THEORY OF NURSING: PRACTICAL APPLICATION

Christine M Chapman OBE BSc (HonsSoc) MPhil SRN SCM RNT FRCN

Professor of Nursing Education
Department of Nursing Studies
University of Wales College of Medicine
Cardiff

Harper & Row, Publishers
London

Cambridge
Hagerstown
Philadelphia
New York

San Francisco
Mexico City
São Paulo
Sydney

First published 1985

Harper & Row Ltd
28 Tavistock Street
London WC2E 7PN

British Library Cataloguing in Publication Data

Chapman, Christine M.
Theory of Nursing: practical application.
1. Nursing
I. Title
610-73 RTH

ISBN 0-06.318326-9

Typeset by Gedset Limited, Cheltenham.
Printed and bound by Butler & Tanner Ltd,
Frome and London.

CONTENTS

PREFACE

The stimulus to write this book came initially from my own students, who bemoaned the absence of a British book on theory in nursing. However, when the idea was floated, it appeared that there was an even greater need to be met, that of students in courses leading to initial registration. Hence the level of presentation. It is hoped that as an introductory text it will whet the appetite of readers for more and, in particular, that they will go to the original publications, hence the section on further reading.

The small practical exercises are meant to encourage readers to apply the theory, not just to read about it.

ACKNOWLEDGEMENTS

Thanks must go to students and staff of the Department of Nursing Studies, University of Wales College of Medicine, for their help and encouragement in the preparation of the book. However, the responsibility of the material included within it is mine.

Special thanks to my secretary, Mrs Eileen Webb, for her skill in reading my handwriting and translating it into readable typescript.

PART I

WHAT IS THEORY?

CHAPTER ONE

DEVELOPMENT OF THEORY

No one seriously disputes that nursing is essentially a practical activity. While the popular image of the nurse soothing a fevered brow may be a romantic and inaccurate picture, nevertheless, when members of the public are asked to describe nursing, they provide descriptions of nurses 'doing' things such as making beds, taking temperatures, giving bedpans, and so on. Even if the type of nursing specified is that related to the mentally ill or handicapped, a list of activities is still mentioned, although of a different nature, such as helping the patient carry out normal living activities, training in social skills, or teaching simple tasks. Therefore, if all agree on the practical nature of nursing, what is meant by nursing theory and what is its function? Does it have any relevance for the nurse in the day-to-day bustle of the ward, or in pressure to provide care in the community, or in prevention and health education?

The aim of this book is to answer these questions and it is important at the start to ensure that author and reader share the same understanding of the words used. In particular, three main terms which form the foundation of the rest of the chapters need definition. These are concept, theory and model.

Concept

This is an abstract notion or idea, often conveyed by a single word, although the features of the concept may be extremely complex. Consider, for example, the breadth and depth of ideas that are conveyed in the words 'health', 'care', 'homeostasis', 'body image' or the 'family'. To take the concept of 'the family', this stimulates mental pictures of relationships such as father, mother, brother, sister, child, parent. In some countries, or indeed in the UK, but in different cultures, the relationships will also include grandparents, aunts, uncles, cousins. However, 'the family' may also convey the feeling of security, the place where everything is alright, or alternatively a feeling of oppression and restriction; an idea of love or of vendetta. Indeed, in some cases in Western countries, the term may be used in a way that is contradictory to the basic idea behind the concept. For example, it is possible to talk of a 'one parent family'.

So, in everyday life we use terms which act as a form of shorthand in conveying meaning. Concepts which imply far more than the dictionary definition of the word, instead representing a range of interacting ideas which are likely to be different in different cultures.

Theory

Theory may be described as a proposed explanation of an event or series of happenings, often demonstrating the relationship of one concept with another. Indeed, concepts may be said to be the building bricks of theory. Theories may, or may not, be proven. A theory which is advanced as an explanation of a happening is more accurately called a 'hypothesis'. This may be stated in varying ways: positively, as in the statement: 'When A occurs, then B will also occur'. A common example of this is when one states that there is 'no smoke without fire'. It may be stated negatively, 'There is no relationship between A and B', which could be demonstrated by the statement that squint is not related to the colour of the person's eyes. It is the job of the researcher to test such hypotheses. This is done by investigating a large number of incidence relating to the hypothesis (the sample) and analysing how often the stated relationship does, or does not, occur (correlation). Statistical tests then have to be applied to ensure that any relationship could not have occurred by chance, in order to show that the findings are significant. Providing the investigation is carried out in such a manner that bias is eliminated, then the original hypothesis may be said to be proved, or not proved. It is important, however, to remember that a theory is only proven at a given state of knowledge and may later be shown to be false. For many years it was held that the atom was the smallest unit of matter, then Cockcroft and fellow workers found a way to split it!

Model

A model is a representation of reality. This is a tool used in many walks of life to enable a real situation to be understood, even when it is not able to be experienced. An obvious and simple example is that of a child's model car which enables a child to feel, to a small extent, what it may be like to drive a car. A model is therefore a representation of reality, frequently abstract, which contains many, or most, of the features of reality but is *not* real.

Models may be pictorial, one-, two- or three-dimensional, structural or abstract. A good example of a pictorial type of model is the London Underground map which shows the relationship of the different lines to each other, the order in which stations occur, where it is possible to change from one line to another, and whether the line is going north, south, east or west. As such, it is used extensively as a guide, enabling thousands of people a day to get about London and its suburbs, yet the map is nothing like reality. In fact, none of the lines run completely straight, but bend and wind their way underground. There is no indication of the depth underground that the trains run, or indeed when they cease to run beneath the earth and surface. There is no actual distance between the stations specified and the relative gaps are somewhat arbitrary, but it fulfils its purpose as a model in that it enables people to understand the complex reality of the London Underground system in such a way that they are able to utilize it to their benefit.

At the other end of the scale are the three-dimensional models beloved by architects and town planners. These can frequently be seen in estate agents' windows as small houses placed along tiny roads, trees, lawns, shops, schools, all in a pattern which is said to represent the final appearance of a new housing estate. Prospective buyers, by studying the model, can decide whether they want a house next to a bus stop, near the shops, or overlooking a field. No one claims that the houses will look exactly like those in the model, or that the trees will be a symmetrical cone shape, but the feature is sufficiently near reality to aid understanding and to enable an informed decision to be made with regard to the future living environment.

In nursing, most models used are of the first type: two-dimensional drawings which show the relationships of variables and enable lines of action to be seen in much the same way as the lines of the Underground may be followed. Such models may act as a tool to enable nursing action to be studied in some cases, to enable the outcome of action to be predicted.

Many people feel that the isolation of concepts, the proving and testing of theory and the formation and use of models is an unnecessary complication in the busy life of the nurse. All that is needed is that the nurse does what she is told, sticks to routine and gets on with the tasks. This type of working, however, is unintelligent and based on the assumption that all patients are alike and that once a patient with a specific medical condition has been cared for, then all subsequent patients with the same condition can be cared for in the same way. Equally, the care of the patient is seen as a series of independent tasks and at no point is the patient conceived of as an indivisable, ideosyncratic, unique person. Action is also taken without certainty of outcome and much care is based on trial and error, which is expensive in time and potentially dangerous to the patient. The use of theory, which can be used as a framework for action, helps to eliminate this random type of care by enabling the nurse to explain patient need and behaviour, to plan to meet those requirements and to predict the likely outcome of nursing interaction. The use of a model may help to order and operationalize the theory so that all care may be rational and specific for the individual patient and particular situation.

This is not as new as it sounds for two reasons:

1 Florence Nightingale used a theory in that she believed that the patient had to recover from his illness by the activity of his own body (in the days of no antibiotics, limited anaesthesia and embryonic medical knowledge, what else could happen?) She therefore stated that the function of the nurse was to control the patient's environment and to provide adequate nourishment so that the patient would be aided in his own recovery.

   Her theory was similar to many used today and indicates that action must be purposeful and focused if care is to be effective.

2 Many of the tasks performed by nurses are based on theory. Not nursing theory, but theory from other disciplines. Every time a patient's temperature is taken, the laws of thermodynamics are used. Every time a wound is dressed using an aseptic technique, the laws based on germ theory are used. When a health visitor calls at a home to assess the progress of a baby, theories of child development are utilized. The list is endless.

In other situations, nursing tasks are performed in a specific way because the effectiveness of that method has been demonstrated, sometimes in a laboratory far removed from a patient, sometimes in a similar clinical situation. The care of patient is, however, more than the performance of a series of tasks, the patient is an indivisible whole and so a theory or framework is required to integrate these tasks into a whole coordinated sequence of action.

Perhaps this is the point to consider whether it is reasonable to expect one theory to fit all types of patient in all situations. Such a theory would be described as a 'macro theory'. Probably the development of such an all-encompassing theory is not possible; patients, or clients, do differ in fundamental ways, for example, the mother having ante-natal care, a normal delivery and postnatal period is not sick. Neither is the toddler being assessed by the health visitor. Even patients with a psychiatric disturbance are sick in a different way from the patient with acute appendicitis. It is therefore likely that a different theory will be needed to act as a framework in each of these cases. True, temperature taking, if required, would have the same theoretical background, that is the macro theory may be the same, but a micro theory of nursing applicable to all would have to be so broad and vague that it would be of limited use. However, by the end of the book, the reader may be able to decide whether there can be 'a theory of nursing'.

CHAPTER
TWO

WHERE DOES NURSING THEORY COME FROM?

Deduction

In Chapter 1, it was demonstrated that some theory used by nurses came from other disciplines. Sometimes such theory is used in very much the same way as originally stated. In other cases it is deduced that the theory developed in one situation can be applied to nursing. For example, the theories from physics related to cooling, state, that as heat is taken from a body to achieve evaporation of water so the body is cooled. This can be used to understand the action of sweating and to substantiate the usefulness of tepid sponging in reducing a patient's temperature.

Induction

Induction is the activity of producing theory out of nursing practice. Such theory must be able to be tested for its validity and usefulness in nursing practice and, of course, the danger of a circular activity, or bias, due to personal experience must be avoided. Dickoff and James (1972) assert that nursing practice is the alpha and omega of nursing theorizing and research.

How is this done? Dickoff and James (1972) feel that as a practitioner brings existing practice to conceptual awareness, that is theorizing, and most of this discussion on theory formation in nursing is based on an article they wrote in 1968. The fact that routine and tradition are beloved by most nurses indicates that many of them are involved in the first steps in the production of theory, that is *isolating factors* by naming them and then placing them in categories. The next step of *factor relating* is carried out by describing the factors so that they are clearly recognized and then linking them. Having achieved this stage, it is possible to progress to the next stage, that of *situation relating* so that events may be predicted and either promoted or inhibited and hence, finally, *produce situations.* As stated in Chapter 1, theories produced in this way will need research in order to test whether the theory works in practice and this is the role of the researcher.

So, the production of theory requires the practitioner, the theory builder and the researcher. These may be three separate people, or alternatively one person may function in all these roles. There is a great deal of evidence that many experienced nurses are using particularly methods of care which 'work' for them, hence the often quoted phrase 'Sister likes it done like this', despite methods normally taught or recommended in the local procedure book. This is a fruitful field for research to see if the claim for that method's superiority to any other is justified. If so, it should be adopted, not only locally but throughout the profession.

To demonstrate this process, it may be helpful to take a simple example. Consider the case of a patient with an acute gastro-intestinal infection. The nurse may note that the patient has severe diarrhoea, vomiting and is sweating due to a raised temperature. These factors, having been named, can now be placed in the category of 'fluid loss'. At the same time, the nurse will also notice the patient's dry mouth, sunken eyes, inelastic skin, reduced urinary output, all of which may be listed and then categorized as signs of dehydration.

The next stage is relating these two categories with each other, ie, fluid loss occurring with dehydration. Once this has been done, it should be possible to predict and take action which will inhibit the onset of dehydration. However, to ensure that this sequence of events is not occurring by chance, research is needed. Possible hypotheses could be as follows:

1 When the fluid lost from the body is in excess of that taken in, then dehydration occurs.

2 Dehydration (as measured by blood concentration) is demonstrated by dry mouth, sunken eyes, inelastic skin and reduced urinary output.

The next step is the collection of a sample of patients with symptoms of fluid loss, recording whether the signs stipulated are present. When a sufficiently large number of cases have been recorded, then the lines on which the proposed correlation occur are stated and a statistical test of significance should be applied to ensure that the correlation has not occurred by chance. Finally, the hypotheses may be said to be proved or disproved. Diagramatically, the process is as shown in Figure 2.1

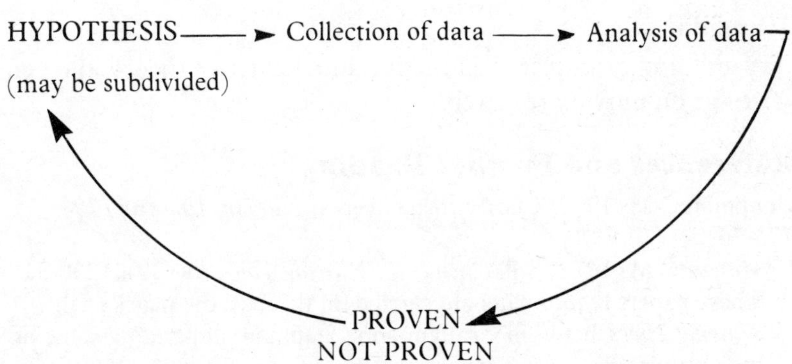

Figure 2.1 Steps in the production of theory

Glaser and Strauss (1967) also wrote about the induction of theory from practice. They used the term 'grounded theory' which they say is obtained by observation and comparison that is repeated until extraneous items are excluded. The items left after this constant comparison may be used to formulate hypotheses, or to advance plausible explanations (their term).

Some situations do not lend themselves to the type of research described (called 'positivism' in that it deals with qualifiable facts). Such an approach may not be appropriate when the meaning of actions is under examination. In this case, a description of situations may require analysis in terms of the perceptions of the people involved. Such analysis is called 'phenomenology', that is the understanding of phenomenon that occur when people meet and interact, and may include the study of the language used, facial expressions, etc. Obviously, it is not possible to reproduce any specific situation, each one is unique. The testing of the findings and categories suggested can only be done by the constant observation of a large number of similar interactions. This type of research is particularly useful in nursing, as many of the situations are dependent on understanding the meaning attached to them by the factors involved, ie, the nurse and the patient.

Exercise

Try and find examples of inductive and deductive theory in recent writings on nursing research.

References and Further Reading

Chapman C M (1972) Clarify the concepts. *Nursing Times* **68** (25): 775-76

Chapman C M (1972) Still clarifying. *Nursing Times* **68** (39): 1230-31

These papers record a debate carried on through the pages of the *Nursing Times*, between Graham and Chapman, illustrating some of the arguments used to support nursing theory.

Dickoff J & James P (1968) A theory of theories: a position paper. *Nursing Research* **17** (3): 197-203

This is American in origin and hence initially a little difficult to read. Nevertheless, it is important as it is in America that the development of nursing theory started.

Dickoff J & James P (1972) Theory development in nursing. In *Nursing Research* Verhorick P (ed.). Little, Brown and Co., Boston

See Dickoff & James (1968) for comments

Glaser B & Strauss A (1967) *The Discovery of Grounded Theory: Strategies for Qualitative Research.* Aldine Press, Chicago

See Dickoff & James (1968) for comments.

Graham S (1972) Excuse me Professor, but have you seen my patient? *Nursing Times* **68** (23): 408-10

Graham S (1972) Just clarify. *Nursing Times* **68** (27): 849-50

These papers record a debate carried on through the pages of *Nursing Times,* between Chapman and Graham, illustrating some of the arguments used to support nursing theory.

Jacox A (1974) Theory construction in nursing: an overview *Nursing Research* **23** (1): 4-13

See Dickoff J & James P (1968) for comments.

McFarlane J K (1976) The role of research and development of nursing theory. *Journal of Advanced Nursing* **1** (6): 443-50

Contains an overview of much of the material written on theory development. It has a useful bibliography.

CHAPTER THREE

MODELS IN NURSING

As already stated in Chapter 1, a model is an abstract representation containing many of the features of reality, but it is not real. Its purpose is to act as a tool, or a device, by which the activity, in this case nursing, can be studied. The important requirements of a model, if it is to be of any value, are that it should demonstrate the relationship of one part with another in terms of space or time, and that it should show how movement may occur.

A simple physiological example may help: A rather crude diagram of a heart is shown in Figure 3.1, which shows the relationship of the chambers of the heart and the vessels leaving and entering it. However, Figure 3.1 gives no indication of the relative size of any of the chambers or blood vessels, and no indication of the direction of blood flow. Figure 3.2 rectifies the latter point by a simple addition of arrows showing the direction of blood flow in the heart.

Though Figures 3.1 and 3.2 help in understanding the function of the heart, they leave many essential features of reality unrepresented. Figure 3.3 therefore illustrates a three-dimensional life-size model of the relative size of the chambers, thickness of walls, actual

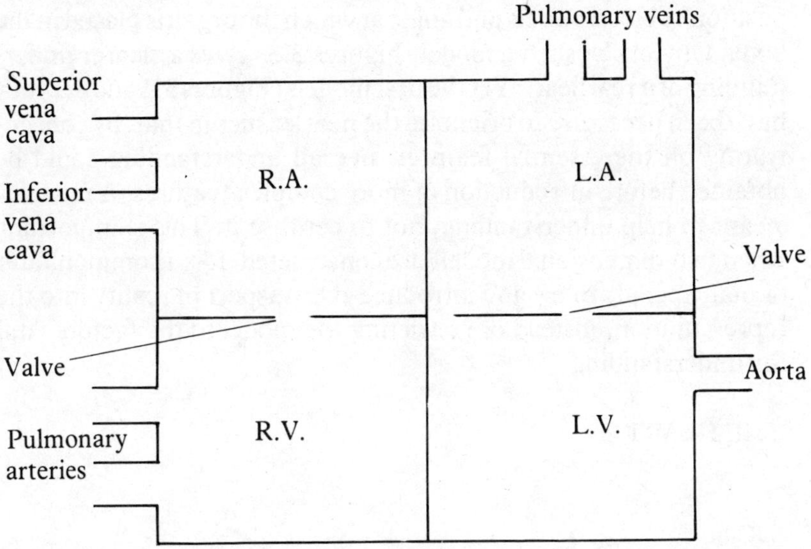

Figure 3.1 A simple model of the heart

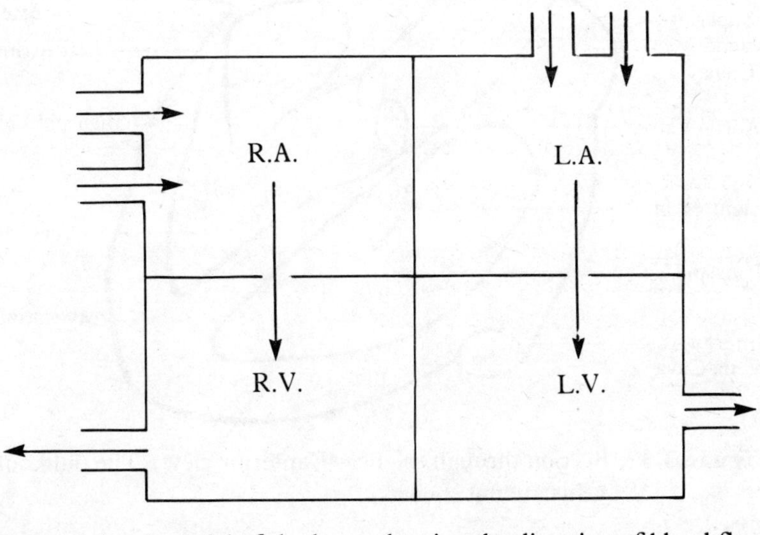

Figure 3.2 A model of the heart showing the direction of blood flow

position of blood vessels and angle at which the organ is placed in the body. Obviously, such a model (Figures 3.3) gives a clearer understanding of a real heart. Yet the first models (Figures 3.1 and 3.2) may have been necessary to orientate the new learner in that, by concentrating on the essential features, overall understanding could be obtained before introduction of more complex features. A model is meant to help understanding, not to confuse it. This is important when two-dimensional models are constructed. It is a common fault of many people to try and introduce every aspect of reality into the representation, instead of restricting the model to the factors vital for understanding.

THE HEART

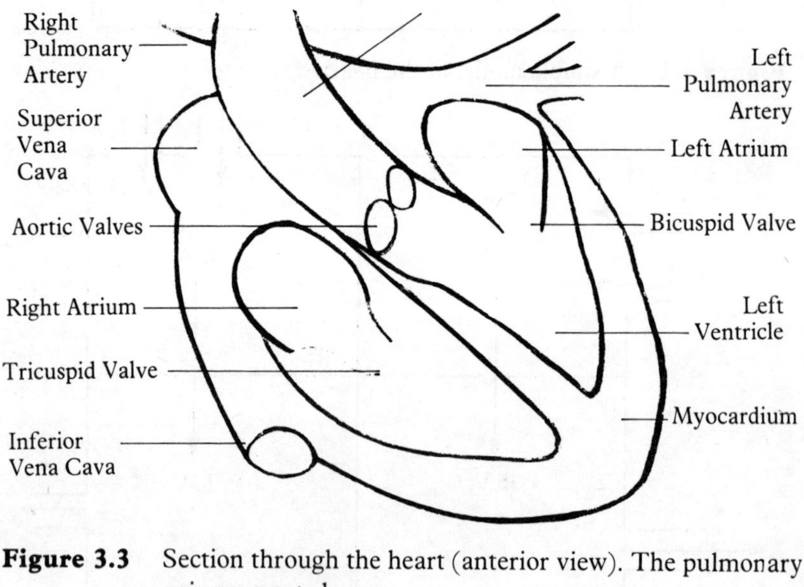

Figure 3.3 Section through the heart (anterior view). The pulmonary veins are not shown

Consider the two models of fluid balance shown in Figure 3.4. While the first model may be more accurate and produce more information, the second is easier to understand and immediately conveys the intended message. Elaboration can take place once initial understanding has been achieved.

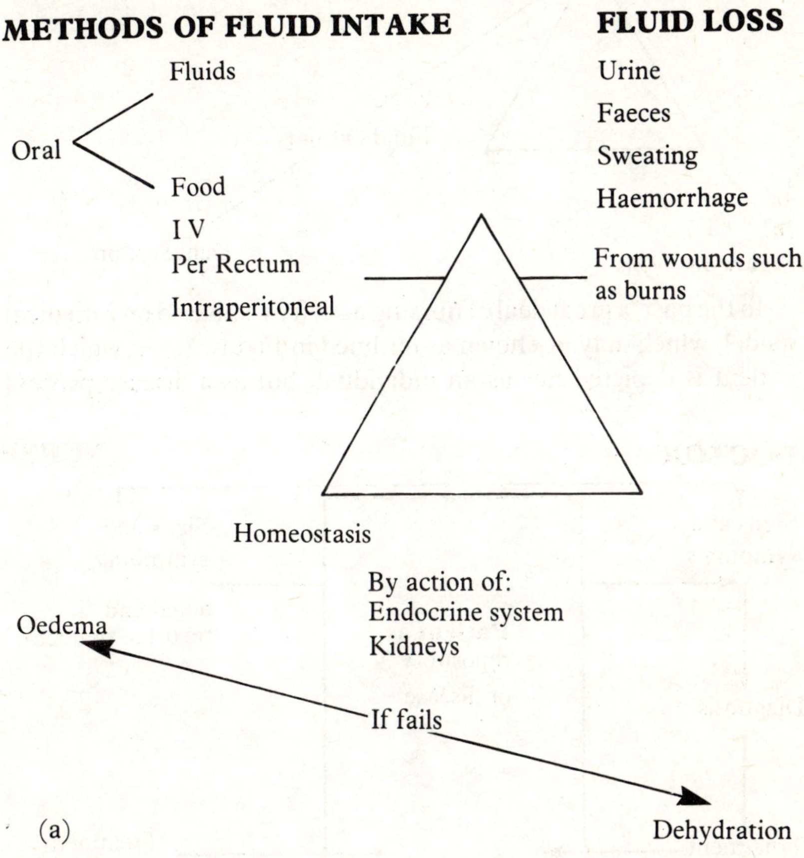

Figure 3.4 Two models of fluid balance: detailed (a) and simplified (b)

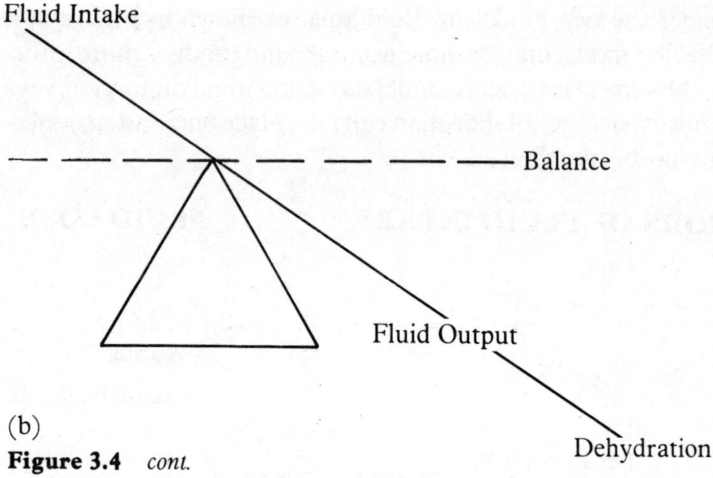

(b)

Figure 3.4 *cont.*

In the past, a great deal of nursing activity was based on a medical model, which may be shown as outlined in Figure 3.5 in which the patient is depicted not as an individual, but as a disease process

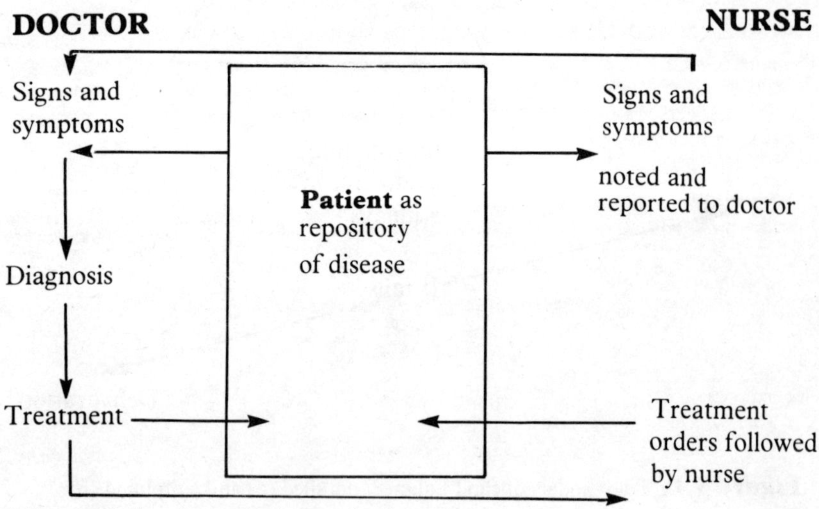

Figure 3.5 A medical model of nursing

exhibiting signs and symptoms. The nurse is seen as the recorder of these signs and symptoms, passing the information to the doctor, who uses them to make a diagnosis and orders treatment, most of which is carried out by the nurse. Such a model does not allow for independent nursing action, yet has been frequently followed in both nursing service and education.

Exercise

Take a nursing activity and, by using a two-dimensional model, show how you would explain it to a person with no nursing or medical knowledge.

Author's Comments

Check your model.
Does it show essential features of the activity?
Can you clearly see the relationship of these features in time and/or space?
Is there any indication of function as shown by movement? (Refer to Figure 3.2).

Another Example of a Model

This example shows the use of information when admitting a patient (Figure 3.6). Information goes *into* records and comes *out of* records.

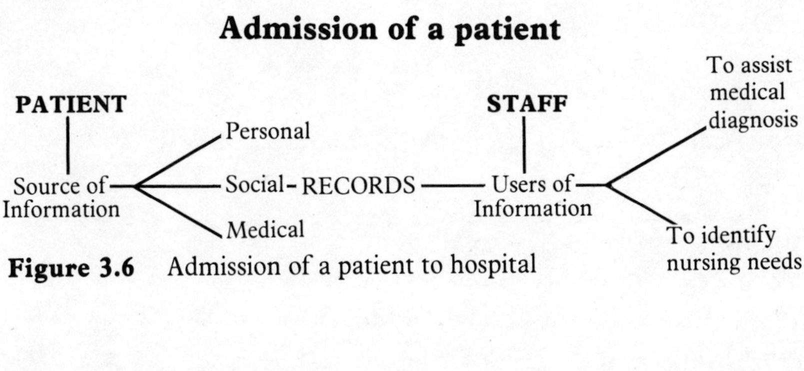

Figure 3.6 Admission of a patient to hospital

Further Reading

Fawcett J (1984) *Analysis and Evaluation of Conceptual Models of Nursing.* F.A. Davis Co., Philadelphia

A comprehensive survey of most models available to date. Advance reading models are tested for their usefulness.

O'Hare E (1980) The gingerbread man. *Nursing Times* **76** (8) 318-20

A simple model to assist in the assessment of patient needs.

Riehl J P & Roy C (1974) *Conceptual Models for Nursing Practice.* Appleton-Century-Crofts, New York.

American text, and rather difficult to read.

Roper N (1976) A model for nursing and nursology. *Journal of Advanced Nursing* **1** (3): 219-27

An early discussion on the use of activities of daily living as a framework for care.

PART II

SPECIFIC THEORIES

CHAPTER FOUR

SYSTEMS

Any organised activity can be described as a system and therefore many theories discussed in future chapters could be included under this heading. However, it is intended here to restrict the discussion to the original concepts as first developed in industry.

Any manufacturing process may be as shown in Figure 4.1: raw materials enter the factory, processing takes place and the outcome is a saleable article.

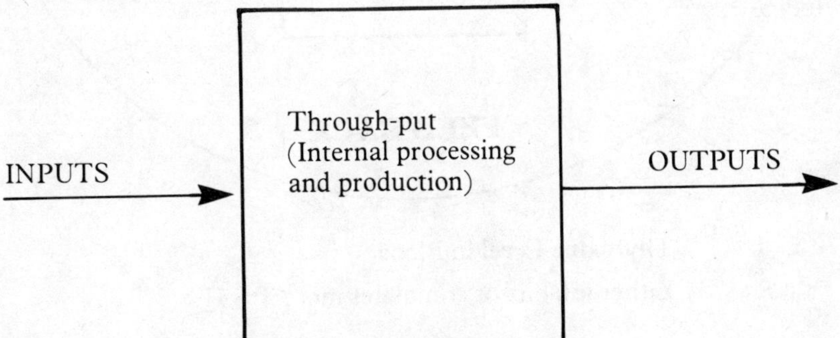

Figure 4.1 An open system of production

In more complex activities, a series of these models may be put together and considered as subsystems (Figure 4.2), as the output from one stage of production becomes an input of another (consider the production of parts for cars which eventually are assembled to become a total car).

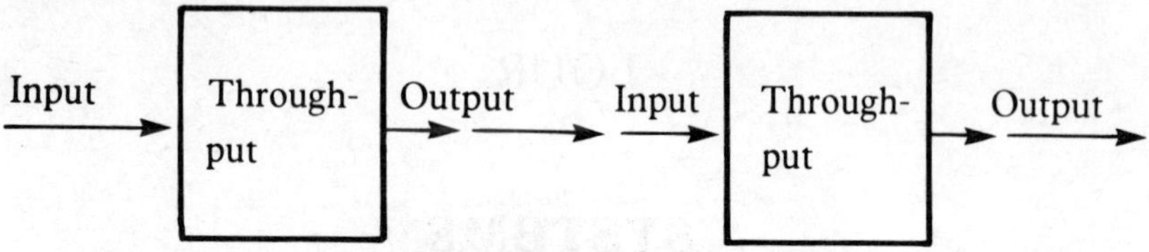

Figure 4.2 A series of open systems of production

Alternatively, in certain cases, the output may act as a moderator of future inputs by means of a feedback mechanism, which is given the term 'cybernetic control'. An excellent example of this type of mechanism is that of the endocrine system. In this model (Figure 4.3), the production of thyroxine from the thyroid gland is demonstrated.

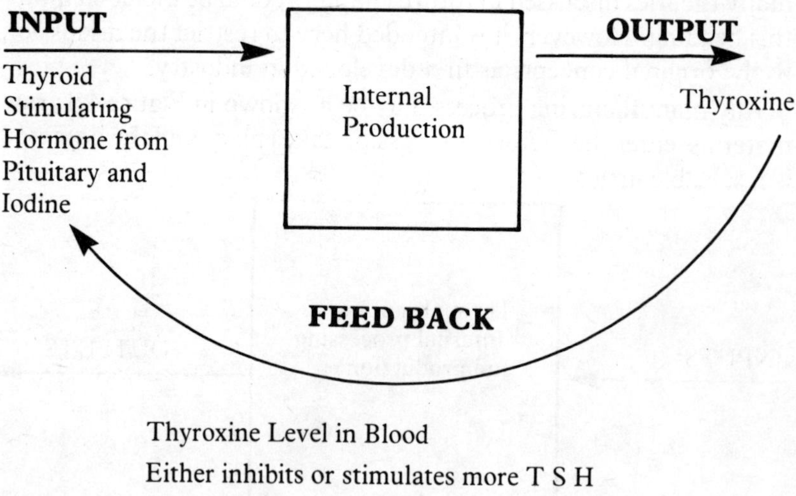

Figure 4.3 The production of thyroxine

Systems may either be 'open', that is able to be influenced by external factors such as the environment, or, in rather rarer situations, 'closed', in that all external factors are excluded. An example of the latter could be the production of certain drugs. This may have to be carried out in a sterile atmosphere with carefully controlled temperature and humidity. In this case, the model would be enclosed (Figure 4.4).

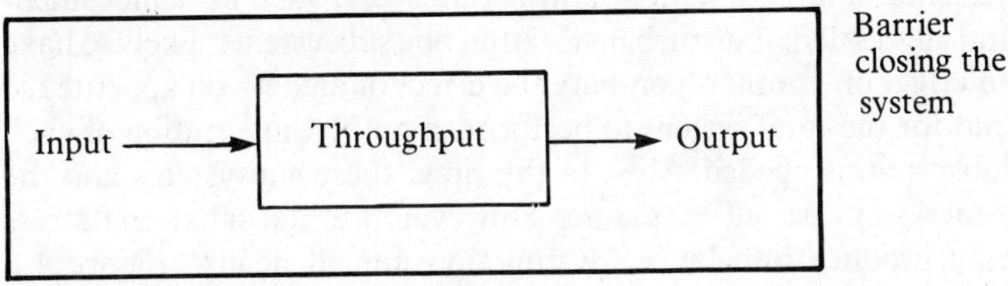

Figure 4.4 A closed system of production

All system models have certain characteristics and assumptions which may be most easily described by referring to the industrial example.

1 The parts must be integrated so that the flow is smooth. Compare the steady movement of an assembly line in a factory. This ensures that the speed of production is maintained to account for the rate at which material can be fed in as input, and allows sufficient time for any activity needed on the journey through the manufacturing process. Equally, it has to take into account the level of output, which should be sufficient to meet demand and perhaps a small stock in reserve, but not result in shortages or an excess in the market. (The latter two factors may act as 'feedback' controls to the process.)

2 They are subject to tension, stress and conflict between the parts. In industry this could be in the form of industrial action, or a machinery breakdown, or it could be the result of external factors, particularly if the boundary is breached.

This system model has been taken up by various nurse theorists. Over many years Dorothy Johnson (1980) developed the idea that man is a behavioural system, with specific response patterns which form an organized and integrated whole. She stated 'All patterned, repetitive and purposeful ways of behaving that characterize men's life can be considered to comprise his behavioural system'. Within this overall functioning are subsystems: physiological such as digestion and elimination, and psychosocial such as achievement and aggression. A disturbance within one subsystem is likely to have an effect on another (compare the effect of anxiety on appetite) so that for the total system to perform smoothly, integration of each subsystem is needed. Most of the time, these subsystems and the total system are self-regulating. However, internal or external stress may produce imbalance, dysfunction and ill health. Figure 4.5 indicates the possible progress of a patient with a wound infection by showing the patient as the unit of production, ie, the place of 'throughput' (Figure 4.1), and demonstrates the physiological changes taking place as a result of the infection. The original input is the infection, but subsequent inputs are the consequence of outputs. These outputs are physical and psychological and are the result of the activity within the body.

Such a model (Figure 4.5) can be used in a variety of ways. It may help explain the sequence of events and thus indicate the reasons for specific actions. This understanding will also help to indicate where intervention by either the nurse and/or the doctor may help break the chain of events and prevent further deterioration, and speed recovery. For example, nursing intervention at the first level of outputs may help relieve pain, eg, steps such as local application of heat to the affected part and elevation, if possible, to help reduce oedema. The doctor's intervention may consist of the ordering of antibiotics to help in the internal struggle against the infection. Later, the nurse may be able to relieve some of the stress exacerbated by pain and fear and help maintain the body so that it can continue its physiological fight.

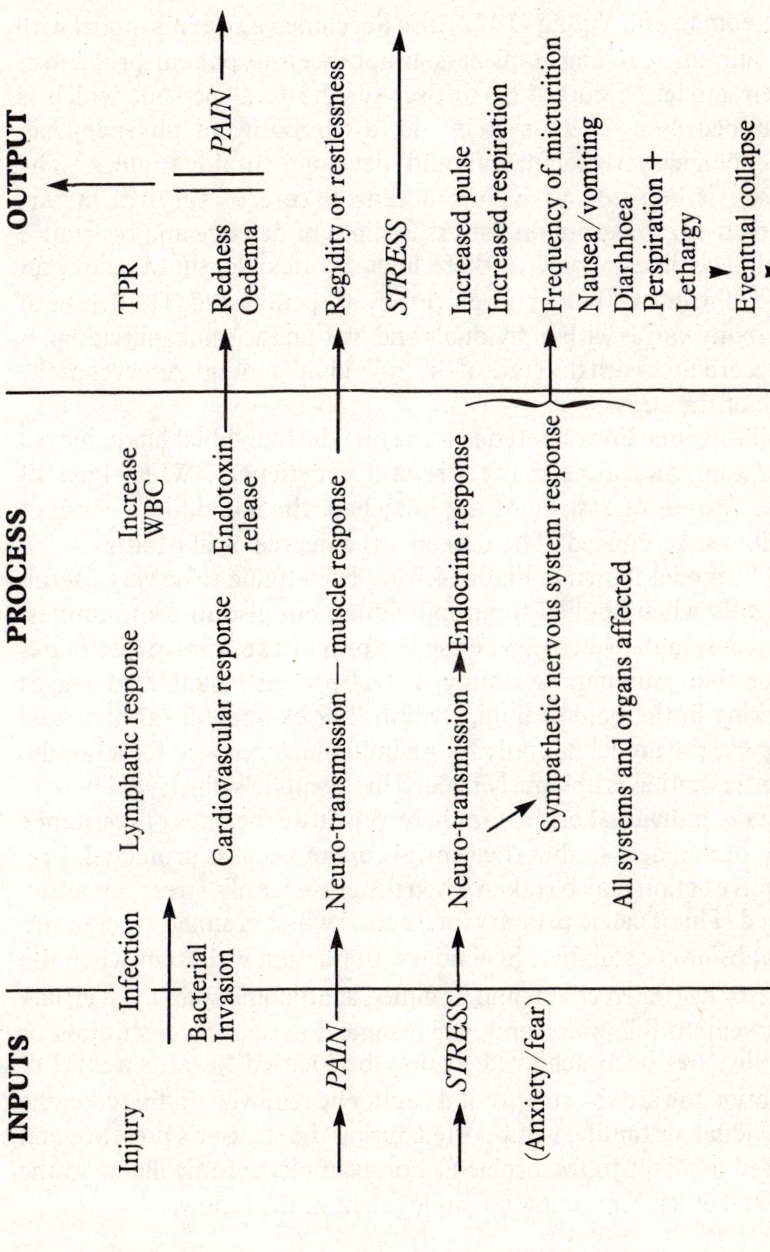

Figure 4.5 The patient as a system

Neuman and Young (1972) also developed a systems model with the aim of 'teaching total person approach to patient problems'. Their model (Figure 4.6) focuses on the total person, which is described as a 'client system', ie, a composite of physiological, psychological, sociocultural and developmental variables. The person is depicted as having a central core of survival factors protected from strain and stress by lines of defence and resistance (boundary lines), some of these lines are flexible, that is they can yield to stressors for a time before they are penetrated. The degree of flexibility varies with individuals and, within the same individual, is in accordance with the state of the individual's energy reserves at the time of the stress.

The normal line of defence is the one the individual has achieved over time and after many stressful experiences. When lines of defence and/or resistance are breached, the individual's sense of 'wellness' is reduced. The outcome is a degree of ill health.

The model shown in Figure 4.7 has been found to be very useful, not only when applied to an individual, but also to communities. Neuman claims that it can be used by providers of care in disciplines other than nursing. Certainly, it has proved valuable to nurses working in the field of public health. For example, health visitors may use the model not only for an individual, but also for a family.

Intervention is obviously needed in the models illustrated here to help the individual or the family reconstitute the lines of resistance and/or defence, so that the central core of needs is protected. Preemptive action may be taken when the presence of a stressor is anticipated. This is called primary interaction which is aimed at retaining equilibrium or stability. Secondary interaction will occur when the stressor has taken effect, and be aimed at attaining stability. Tertiary intervention follows second, when some degree of reconstitution or stability has been achieved. It may be focused towards a level of adaption toward the stressor if it cannot be removed. In this case, the individual, or family, is supported during the stressor's presence and helped to adapt to the problem. For example, chronic illness in the individual, or continuing unemployment in the family.

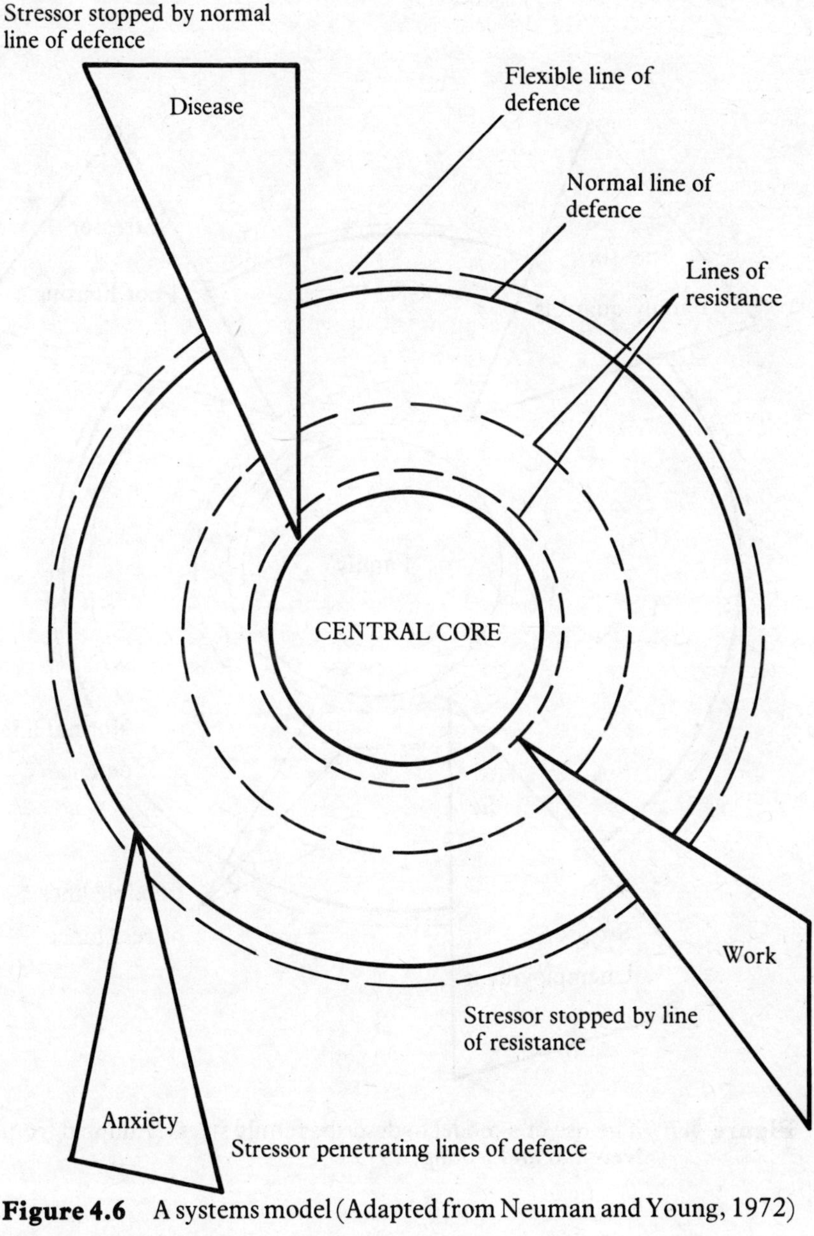

Figure 4.6 A systems model (Adapted from Neuman and Young, 1972)

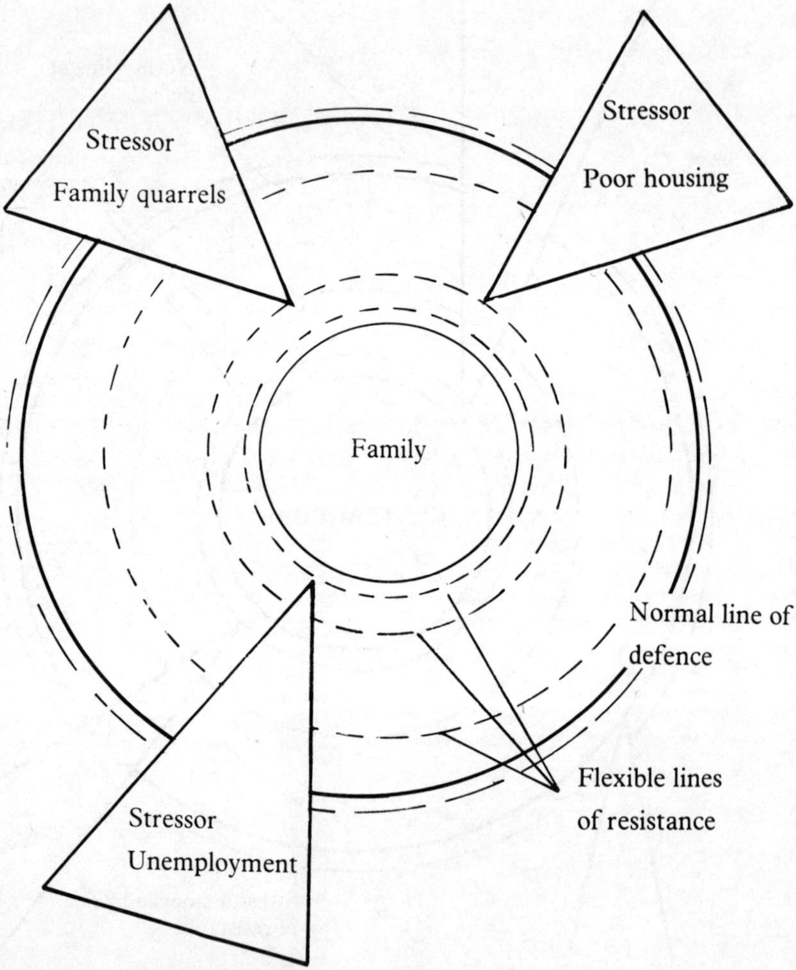

Figure 4.7 The use of a model to describe family stress (Adapted from Neuman and Young, 1972)

Exercise

A 62-year-old lady is admitted to hospital with a lump in her breast and severe pain in the right hip due to osteo-arthritis. Her husband, who is older than her, is blind and will be living alone during her time in hospital.

Using Neuman's model, indicate the likely stressors that will affect this lady, and the way in which the nurse may intervene.

Author's comments

The strength of each of the stressors: lump in breast, pain in hip, anxiety about husband, can only be determined by individual assessment. The nurse may expect the lump, with its possible implications of cancer, to be the most stressful, while in fact continuous pain or anxiety may be more distressing to the patient.

Intervention will focus on each of these factors and will require the activity of other health care team members, such as the doctor and the social worker.

References and Further Reading

Johnson D E (1980) The behavioural system model for nursing, In *Conceptual Models for Nursing Practice*, 2nd ed. Riehl J P & Roy C. Appleton-Century-Crofts, New York.

Johnson (1980) presents in detail the behavioural system model for nursing, and the way in which it may be used in nursing service, education and research. This is the only publication of this model by Johnson, although she discusses it elsewhere.

Neuman B & Young R J (1972) A model for teaching total person approach to patient problems. *Nursing Research* **21**: 265

Neuman and Young (1972) present the original statement of the model for teaching total person approach to patient problems.

Neuman B (1982) *The Neuman Systems Model: Application to Nursing Education and Practice.* Appleton-Century-Crofts, New York.

As stated, Neuman (1982) demonstrates the use of the model in nursing education

CHAPTER
FIVE

ADAPTION

Chapter 4 demonstrated the need for integration and balance within a system, if it is to perform efficiently. This need for equilibrium is well demonstrated in physiology and termed 'homeostasis'. To take a well known example, the body's response to bleeding (Figure 5.1). The balance is controlled automatically by the body using a feedback mechanism. In fact, in life, balance is not a steady state but is dynamic so that there is a constant change from balance to imbalance, back to balance and so on.

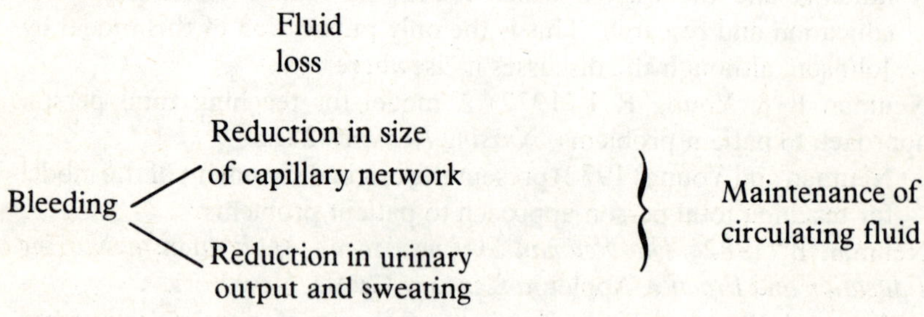

Figure 5.1 The body's response to bleeding

This raises the question, what factors cause imbalance? The answer is comparatively simple: any event which makes a demand on the individual, that is any form of stress, whether it be physiological or psychosocial, internal in origin, or external, will cause imbalance.

Stress is, however, difficult to measure in that the individual's perception of the demand will vary and imbalance will only occur when the individual is unable to meet the demand. Many of us are aware of the fact that sitting an examination is stressful to some extent. However, one candidate will apparently be relatively unconcerned, while another will not be able to sleep or eat prior to the testing day.

Demands, or stressors, can be anything that is experienced in life and a person who is in a chronically stressed condition is in a state of perpetual activity as they try to maintain equilibrium. Such a state may eventually lead to a breakdown in the body's ability to regain balance. When this occurs, illness results to act as a further stressor.

This ability of the body to regain balance, or, to use common language, 'to cope' in the face of stress has been described by Selye (1976) in his General Adaption syndrome (Figure 5.2). However, some diseases are the result of maladaption.

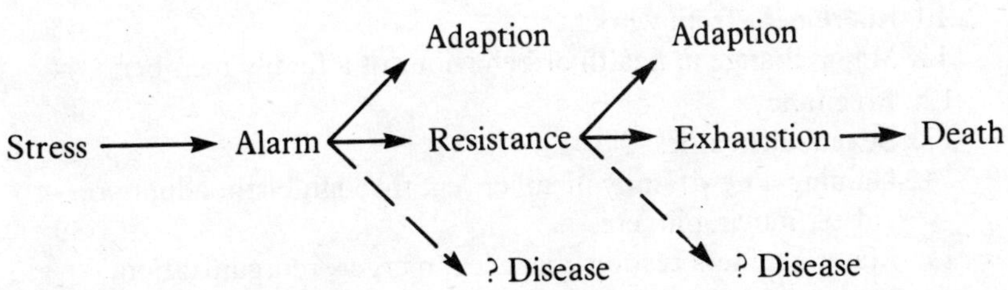

Figure 5.2 The general adaption syndrome (Adapted from Selye, 1976)

Holmes and Rahe (1967) have identified 43 life events which produce stress. By questioning a number of people, they were able to assign a score to each of these events, indicating how stressful they were to this research sample. The base-line used was marriage, that is each respondent was asked to state, in comparison with their marriage, how stressful were the other events. These results were then scaled, with the most stressful being given 100 points (Table 5.1).

Table 5.1 Stress ratings for life events (From Holmes and Rahe, 1967 and reproduced with kind permission of the authors and publishers, Pergamon).

Life Event	Value
1. Death of spouse	100
2. Divorce	73
3. Marital separation from partner	65
4. Detention in jail or other institution	63
5. Death of a close family member	63
6. Major personal injury or illness	53
7. Marriage	50
8. Being fired at work	47
9. Marital reconciliation with partner	45
10. Retirement from work	45
11. Major change in health or behaviour of a family member	44
12. Pregnancy	40
13. Sexual difficulties	39
14. Gaining a new family member (eg, through birth, adoption, oldster moving in, etc.)	39
15. Major business readjustment (eg, merger, reorganization, bankruptcy, etc.)	39
16. Major change in financial state (eg, a lot worse off or a lot better off than usual)	38
17. Death of a close friend	37

Life Event	Value
18. Changing to a different line of work	36
19. Major change in the number of arguments with spouse (eg, either a lot more or a lot less than usual regarding child-rearing, personal habits, etc.)	35
20. Taking out a mortgage or loan for a major purchase (eg, for a home, business, etc.)	31
21. Foreclosure on a mortgage or loan	30
22. Major changes in responsibilities at work, (eg, promotion, demotion, lateral transfer)	29
23. Son or daughter leaving home (eg, marriage, attending college, etc.)	29
24. Trouble with in-laws	29
25. Outstanding personal achievement	28
26. Wife beginning, or ceasing, work outside the home	26
27. Beginning or ceasing formal schooling	26
28. Major change in living conditions (eg, building a new home, remodelling, deterioration of home or neighbourhood)	25
29. Revision of personal habits (dress, manners, association, etc.)	24
30. Troubles with the boss	23
31. Major change in working hours or conditions	20
32. Change in residence	20
33. Changing to a new school	20
34. Major change in usual type and/or amount of recreation	19
35. Major change in church activities (eg, a lot more or a lot less than usual)	19
36. Major change in social activities (eg, clubs, dancing, movies, visiting, etc.)	18
37. Taking out a mortgage or loan for a lesser purchase (eg, for a car, TV, freezer, etc.)	17
38. Major change in sleeping habits (a lot more or a lot less sleep or change in part of day when asleep)	16
39. Major change in number of family get-togethers (eg, a lot more or a lot less than usual)	15

Life Event	Value
40. Major change in eating habits (a lot more or a lot less food intake, or very different meal hours or surroundings)	15
41. Vacation	13
42. Christmas	12
43. Minor violations of the law (eg, traffic tickets, jaywalking, disturbing the peace, etc.)	11

If the list shown in Table 5.1 is studied, it will become apparent that several of the events may occur to one individual simultaneously. For example, marriage (50), taking out a mortgage (31), major change in living conditions (25), recreation (19), social activities (19). If this happens, then the points should be added together, which results in a total score of 144, indicating quite a high level of stress. Holmes and Rahe (1967) felt that a score of over 200 indicated a level of stress which was likely to be too great for the individual's normal coping mechanism. It will be noted that many of the life events on the list are the frequent concern of nurses, eg, bereavement, illness and injury, change in eating habits.

In addition, a further scale (Volicer and Bohannon 1975) has been developed which specifies specifically the order of stress likely to be experienced by patients in hospital. In this scale (Table 5.2), the ranking is different. Number 1 is the least stressful, while number 49 is the most stressful event.

The list shown in Table 5.2 should make all nurses alert to the stressful nature of some events which they may consider unimportant. Note the high ranking of lack of information (37,43 and 44); the staff being in much too much hurry (26); having cold and tasteless food (21). Adding these events to those which have already occurred and which may have helped to produce the illness for which the patient has been admitted to hospital, demonstrates the very high level of stress with which the patients have to live.

Table 5.2 Stress ratings related to hospitalization. (From Volicer and Bohannon 1975, and reproduced with kind permission of the authors and publishers, The American Journal of Nursing Company).

Assigned Rank and Event
1. Having strangers sleep in the same room with you.
2. Having to eat at different times than you usually do.
3. Having to sleep in a strange bed.
4. Having to wear a hospital gown.
5. Having strange machines around.
6. Being awakened in the night by the nurse.
7. Having to be assisted with bathing.
8. Not being able to get newspapers, radio or TV when you want them.
9. Having a room-mate who has too many visitors.
10. Having to stay in bed or the same room all day.
11. Being aware of unusual smells around you.
12. Having a room-mate who is seriously ill or cannot talk with you.
13. Having to be assisted with a bedpan.
14. Having a room-mate who is unfriendly.
15. Not having friends visit you.
16. Being in a room that is too cold or too hot.
17. Thinking your appearance might be changed after hospitalization.
18. Being in the hospital during holidays or special family occasions.
19. Thinking you might have pain because of surgery or test procedures.
20. Worrying about your spouse being away from you.
21. Having to eat cold or tasteless food.
22. Not being able to call family or friends on the phone.
23. Being cared for by an unfamiliar doctor.
24. Being put in hospital because of an accident.
25. Not knowing when to expect things will be done to you.

Assigned Rank and Event

26. Having the staff be in too much of a hurry.
27. Thinking about losing income because of your illness.
28. Having medications cause you discomfort.
29. Having nurses or doctors talk too fast, or use words you can't understand.
30. Feeling you are getting dependent on medications.
31. Not having family visit you.
32. Knowing you have to have an operation.
33. Being hospitalized far away from home.
34. Having a sudden hospitalization you weren't planning to have.
35. Not having your call light answered.
36. Not having enough insurance to pay for your hospitalization.
37. Not having your questions answered by the staff.
38. Missing your spouse.
39. Being fed through tubes.
40. Not getting relief from pain medications.
41. Not knowing the results or reasons for your treatment.
42. Not getting pain medication when you need it.
43. Not knowing for sure what illness you have.
44. Not being told what your diagnosis is.
45. Thinking you might lose your hearing.
46. Knowing you have serious illness.
47. Thinking you might lose a kidney or some other organ.
48. Thinking you might have cancer.
49. Thinking you might lose your sight.

Nursing intervention is aimed at the prevention and reduction of stress. Often the first step is assisting the patient to recognise what events are stressful so that they may be either avoided, or methods of coping prepared. If the stressful events are inevitable, or have already occurred, then the nurse's role is to assist the patient with the adaptive mechanism. Finally, the nurse should also take steps to ensure that none of her actions, or those of her colleagues, contribute to the patient's stress.

Studies by Hayward (1975) and Boore (1978) have shown that the provision of information by a nurse prior to surgery has the effect of lessening postoperative pain and hastening recovery. These studies are a good example of the way that the removal or lessening of a stressor can contribute to the patient's recovery.

Adaption Theory

A further development in the method of approaching care can be found in the theory proposed by Callista Roy (1974), which she names an 'adaption model'. She stated that a person needs a nurse 'when unusual stresses or weakened coping mechanisms make usual attempts to cope ineffective' (Roy and Roberts, 1981).

Roy viewed health as a continuum:

Maximum wellness ___________ maximum illness

and considered that while it is the physician's goal to move the patient along the line from illness to health, the nurse's role is to promote patient adaption in terms of physiological functioning, self-concept, role performance and interdependence during the stages of health and illness.

> 'The projected outcome (of nursing) is an adapted state in the patient which frees him to respond to other stimuli. This freeing of energy makes it possible for the goal of nursing to contribute to the overall goal of the health team, higher level wellness. When energy is freed from inadequate coping attempts, then it can promote healing and wellness'. (Roy and Roberts, 1981).

As in previous models, emphasis is placed on the totality of the person and on the need for the patient to actively participate in his own adaptive behaviour. Nevertheless, this totality is made up of components identified by Roy (1974) as biological, psychological and social.

Adaption in the biological area of life takes place via an internal subsystem described by Roy as the 'regulator'. This subsystem includes neural, endocrine and psychomotor activity. The second subsystem relates to learning, judgement, emotion and perceptual information processing, and is termed the 'cognator' mechanism. They are linked together by perceptions. To quote Roy (1970) 'The regulator mechanism works mainly through the automatic nervous system to set up a reflex action which readies the person for coping with the stimulus by approach, attack or flight. The cognator identifies, stores and relates stimuli so that symbolic responses can be made. It acts consciously by means of thought and decision and unconsciously through defence mechanisms'.

The activity of adaption is seen in the coping behaviour demonstrated in four areas called 'adaptive modes'; physiological, self-concept, role function and interdependence.

Physiological Mode

Adaption in the physiological mode is related to needs such as nutrition, elimination, fluid and electrolytes, oxygen and circulation, regulation of temperature, the senses, the endocrine system, exercise and rest.

The Self-Concept Mode

The self-concept mode is concerned with the view the individual holds of himself, both physiologically and as a person. It encompasses such self-image pictures as physical appearance, toughness/gentleness, and moral or ethical assessments such as good or evil, all of which go to make up the person's assessment of their own worth, both in their eyes and the eyes of others.

Role Function

Role function focuses on the need to have a place and function in society which conveys certain rights or privileges and also carries with it duties or responsibilities.

Interdependence

Interdependence highlights another aspect of social life; the balance required between dependence and independence in relationship with others.

It is obvious from these descriptions that every individual is constantly adapting throughout life, whether in health or illness. However, it is in illness that the individual may require help to carry out this activity and it is here that the nurse may be able to make a contribution, following an assessment of the patient's needs in each of the four areas described, and in collaboration with the patient, both in assessment and goal-setting.

Example

Consider a brief example of the use of the above model:

> A 52-year-old, self-employed, married man with four children admitted to hospital with severe chest pain diagnosed as having suffered a myocardial infarction. Treatment involved includes analgesia, oxygen and cardiac drugs, light nutritive diet, rest with graduated return to exercise.

Areas requiring adaption

Physiological:

Relief of pain
Related to heart activity and its regulation
Assisted by drugs
Need for oxygen, gradually reduced
Concern with all other systems, eg, diet, elimination, etc.

Role Performance:

Need to hand over business for time
No longer able to support wife and family

Interdependence:

Initial dependance, with gradual return to independence (? not at same level as previously).

Self-concept:

May consider himself useless.
Need to have realistic view of future.

Exercise

Develop the above outline in detail, demonstrating how you would set goals for and with the patient, and indicating nursing care.

Author's Comments

This is an example that not only requires you to consider adaption by the patient, but also by his wife and family.

A similar situation, although not identical, can be found in the book by Randell *et al* (1982), where care is described in detail.

References and Further Reading

Boore J (1978) *Prescription for Recovery.* Rcn Research Series, London
A nursing study into the anxiety produced by surgery and stay in hospital.
Hayward J (1975) *Information against pain.* Rcn Research Series, London
A nursing study into the anxiety produced by surgery and stay in hospital.
Holmes T H & Rahe R H (1967) The social re-adjustment scale. *Journal Psychosomatic Research* **2**: 214
Contains the original discussions on stress.
Randell B Tedrow M P & Van Landingham J (1982) *Adaption Nursing. The*

Roy Conceptual Model Applied. C.V. Mosby Co., St. Louis

This contains a series of papers showing how the conceptual model may be used. The examples cover a wide range of situations and discuss the attitudes and actions of the nurses, as well as the patients and clients.

Riehl J P & Roy C (1980) *Conceptual Models for Nursing Practice*, 2 edn. Appleton-Century-Crofts, New York

Roy C (1974) Adaption: A conceptual framework for nursing, *Nursing Outlook* **18** (3): 42-5

Roy (1970) and Riehl & Roy (1980) are just two of the many books and papers written by Roy on the Adaption Model.

Selye H, ed. (1976) *The Stress of Life.* McGraw Hill Book Co., New York

Contains the original discussions on stress.

Volicer B J & Bohannon M W (1975) A hospital stress rating scale. *Nursing Research* **2**: 358

Contains original discussions on stress.

Wilson-Barnett J (1978) Patients' emotional response to barium X-rays. *Journal of Advanced Nursing* **3** (I): 37-45

A nursing study into the anxiety produced by procedures and stay in hospital.

CHAPTER SIX

INTERACTION

Despite the increasing complexity of medical and nursing techniques, which often serve to emphasize nursing tasks, in the final analysis of the question 'What is Nursing?', most people would agree that at the point of delivery of care it is essentially a social activity, an interaction process between two individuals, the nurse and the patient. Even when a group of patients are cared for by a team of nurses, the actual task is one where individuals react with individuals. The unit, then, is two people and what happens when they meet. It is interesting to note that Timasheff (1966) uses virtually the same definition when introducing the study of sociology. If sociology and nursing share a similar definition, it is likely that the study of the one may provide insights into the other, and that sociological theories may contribute to the development of theory in nursing.

This is certainly true when studying interaction in nursing, which owes much to the work of symbolic interactionists such as Mead (1934) and, more recently, Blumer (1964). The latter defines symbolic interaction as that which occurs between human beings who interpret or define each other's actions, instead of just reacting to them.

Imogene King (1971) developed a nursing model using these ideas where she postulated that any nurse-patient encounter could be represented (Figure 6.1). This model demonstrates nursing as a series of incidents which connect action, reaction and interaction, and the transaction that follows when a reciprocal relationship is established between the nurse and the patient participating in the definition of the goal to be achieved. (The fact that the patient may not always be able to participate in this model is appreciated, as is the case in the care of the unconscious patient.)

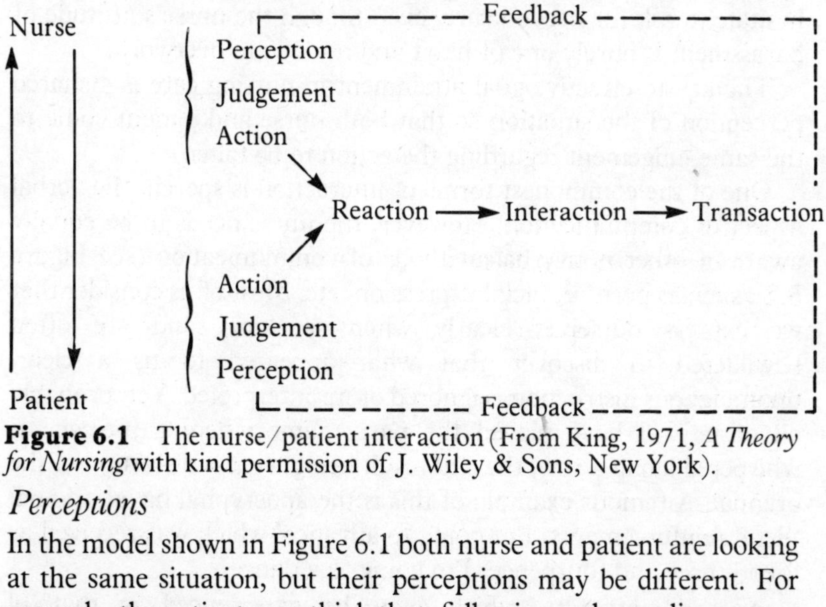

Figure 6.1 The nurse/patient interaction (From King, 1971, *A Theory for Nursing* with kind permission of J. Wiley & Sons, New York).

Perceptions

In the model shown in Figure 6.1 both nurse and patient are looking at the same situation, but their perceptions may be different. For example, the patient may think that, following orthopaedic surgery, his leg should be kept quite still to prevent pain, while the nurse may think that quadriceps muscle exercises will be beneficial: each will act appropriately and a deadlock may occur. However, if both realise that the other is seeing the situation differently, their reactions to the proposed action will result in communication, explanation and understanding, with an appropriate change in the actions of one, or possibly a compromise (eg, the patient will be given analgesics to relieve the discomfort and he will then perform the exercises). This approach emphasises the importance of perception and the fact that nurse and patient may contact each other. However, if benefit is to be produced by this contact, a transaction needs to take place. If the nurse, using her own standards, perceives the patient as 'making a fuss', she will use that as a basis of her actions regardless of whether or not the patient's behaviour can be explained by medical, psychological or cultural facts. Equally, a patient who perceives a nurse as 'too busy' will hesitate to ask for needed care, even though the nurse's attitude of harassment is purely one of habit and not due to overwork.

The key to effective goal attainment in nursing care is a shared perception of the situation so that both nurse and patient come to the same judgement regarding the action to be taken.

One of the commonest forms of interaction is speech, the verbal aspect of communication. However, the nurse needs to be equally aware of other nonverbal methods of communication (see Figure 6.2), such as posture, facial expression, etc. Most of us consider that we express ourselves clearly when speaking, and are often bewildered to discover that what appeared to us a clear, unambiguous instruction is ignored or misinterpreted. Yet, probably all of us will have played the party game where a message is whispered along a row, the end result being a gross distortion of the original. A famous example of this is the apocryphal naval original 'Send reinforcements, I'm going to advance' which was received as 'Send three and fourpence, I'm going to a dance'.

Another difficulty which may be experienced is that of understanding. Words have meaning attached to them, but the meaning must be shared by both the sender of the message and the person receiving it. If a message is sent to me in English, I may be able to understand it. If in Greek, then it may as well not be sent.

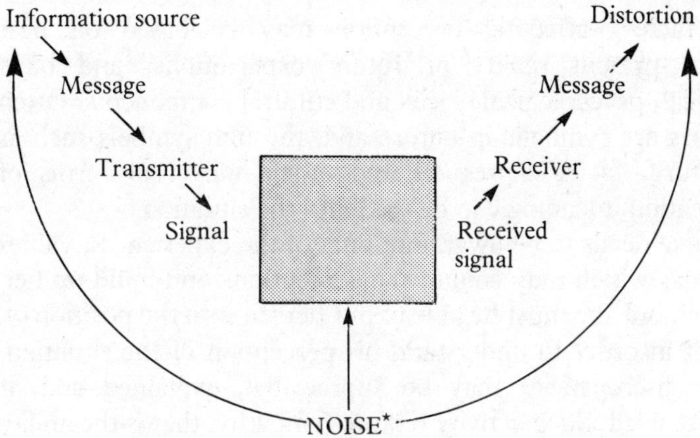

*Noise, in this context, is any factor which may interfere with the signal. For example, it may be actual noise (eg, an electric drill) or, as in the case of a patient, pain or anxiety.

Figure 6.2 A simple model of the communication process

> A small boy visiting Holland with his parents went to join some Dutch children playing outside. Within minutes he was back crying in despair 'They can't hear me and I can't hear them'. Of course none of the children were deaf, but they might as well have been for all the value that they were getting from talking to each other.

Nonverbal communication can be equally problematic. In some cultures and situations, touch may be seen as a friendly supportive gesture, in others as an invasion of personal privacy and a threat. Nurses and doctors, because of their priviledged role, are often allowed to touch people in a way not permitted in normal social interaction. Most patients understand this, but some resent and resist the breaking down of social taboos, which are deeply engrained. The problem of male doctors wishing to care for women in some Moslem countries is well known, but similar problems can be found in many other situations. Communication, verbal and nonverbal, is one way of understanding the perception of another to any given situation.

Other factors affecting perception may be based on past experience, present reality or future expectations, and have physiological, psychological, social and cultural components. Often such factors are symbolic in nature and, through symbols such as body posture, facial expression and other nonverbal forms of communication, meaning can be read into the situation.

The nurse needs to be aware not only of the experiences, values and attitudes which may colour her perceptions and build-up her 'self-image', but she must be able to put herself into the position of the patient in order to understand his perception of the situation. This way discrepancies may be appreciated, explained and, if possible, resolved. Such activity requires empathy, that is the ability to 'stand where he stands'. Obviously, this is easier if the nurse has actually been in the same situation on some occasion, hence the idea that all nurses should have had experience of being a patient! However, it is likely that empathy can be developed by analysis of situations, either at the time or by the use of videotapes of situations and by role play.

There are problems. Previous experience may facilitate or hinder the activity of empathy, and the nurse may not wish to experience empathy or indeed see it to be of value; Singh (1972) suggested that British nurses did not feel a need to develop strong relationships with patients. Emphasis on task performance, the consideration of the patient only as someone to whom something has to be done, or even someone to be studied, are likely to hinder empathy.

Many nurses believe that it is bad to get 'involved' with the patient. A commonly held view is that it is only by being detached that the nurse can carry out tasks for the patient which may be embarrassing if viewed in the context of the culture, may be unpleasant and/or offensive to the nurse, or are painful for the patient. Equally, detachment may be seen as the hallmark of professionalism, so that the neophyte may deliberately dampen any sense of warmth or tenderness, and aim at cold efficiency. In social work, Scott (1966) comments 'case workers, as professionals, were expected to relate to the client in a detached, emotionally neutral manner. The control of emotional affect in relationship with clients is meant to encourage impartial service and to ensure that the practitioner's judgement is guided by reason rather than emotion'. It is the need to apply reasonable judgement that requires the next stage in empathy. Indeed, it is this latter stage of empathy — the withdrawal and critical scrutiny of the situation — that distinguishes the empathy used in a clinical situation from that which occurs spontaneously in everyday life, and this ability to withdraw is the skill that is required in involvement with patients.

Mead (1934) described a similar activity as 'role taking' . That is the symbolic process by which one person puts himself into the other's place to gain insight, anticipate the other's behaviour, and to act accordingly. Thinking is the process by which this activity is conducted. It allows varying paths of action to be explored and rejected before the final one is translated into action, thus cutting short a great deal of 'trial and error' behaviour.

Within this model, therefore, instead of the nurse performing tasks 'on' the patient, with greater or lesser patient cooperation, the nurse and the patient act as a team working towards a common goal.

Judgement

Perception is crucial to judgement. We have all probably had the experience of waiting for one important interview and being put in a waiting room by ourselves, without a clock. Time appears to stand still. The feeling grows that we have been forgotten, until the feeling that we must remind someone that we still exist is overwhelming and we get up and look for a receptionist, who reassures us that we will soon be attended to. A glance at the clock shows that only 30 minutes have passed, not the perceived hours, and therefore our judgement of the perceived fact was faulty and our action unnecessary.

Time certainly is a major factor affecting the perception of patients. Roth, while a patient in a hospital for tuberculosis sufferers described how the patients constructed elaborate ways of marking off time in terms of when they would be allowed out of bed, when they would have specific treatments, or when they would be discharged. The problem was that the resources they used, often comparison with other patients, were inappropriate in their case (Roth, 1963).

To the patient lying in bed with little to do, either because of medical incapacity or lack of motivation, the time between breakfast and lunch may seem endless, while to the hard-pressed nurse it goes in a flash. No wonder that patients resent being told 'in a minute' when making a request to a nurse, or that the nurse is bewildered when the patients complain of the length of time they have been kept waiting. Their judgement is affected by their perception of time and, as Thomas and Znancechi (1927) have said, 'As men perceive a situation to be real, it is real in its consequences' and action is therefore dependent on the judgement of reality regardless of any objective factual measurement.

Actions

The symbolic meanings attached to actions must also be considered. In Britain, it is common practice to offer a visitor a drink, traditionally a cup of tea, although coffee is rapidly taking precedence. This is not because the visitor is physically in need of a drink, but it is a gesture of friendship and hospitality. A similar interpretation may be placed on the cup of tea given to a newly admitted patient. This may be deliberate policy and used as a welcoming token, but more likely it will occur (if it does) by chance in that all patients are being served tea at that time. (Chapter 9 discusses further the symbolic value of actions).

Reaction

So, perception leads to judgement which guides action which, in turn, stimulates a reaction from other people in the situation. This reaction may be one of rejection of the initial action, acceptance in a passive sense in that the action is perceived but not entered into, or it may be a collaborative reaction in which the action by A is welcomed by B and stimulates B's own involvement. It is this collaborative action which is described as interaction leading to an outcome, ie, transaction.

For nurses to achieve any therapeutic relationship with patients, this stage of transaction is essential. The old idea of nurses 'doing things' to patients, the nurse being active and the patient passive, is only legitimate when the patient is unable to participate by reason of age or unconscious. Even the physically incapacitated can participate mentally, and often the mentally disabled will participate physically. The aim is that of a shared goal, one to which both sides are agreed is desirable, relevant and practical. In order for a long term goal to be practical, it may have to be broken down into subsidiary goals, but each step must be agreed upon, as must the methods by which it may be achieved.

The level and success of interaction achieved between the nurse and the patient is one of the critical factors by which quality of nursing care can be measured. While measurement of interaction may seem to be a subjective measure, the affect of the transaction will, or will not, result in the achievement of objective goals.

Exercise

Miss Mary Jones, aged 86, had been a headmistress of a girls' private school in a town in the South of England. During a holiday in the North of England, she developed a high temperature, nausea and frequency of micturition. The doctor called to the small hotel in which she was staying diagnosed a urinary infection. As she could not be cared for in the hotel, she was admitted to the geriatric ward in the District General Hospital. On admission, she was a well-nourished, alert lady, who obviously had high standards of personal cleanliness and appearance. In view of this, the nurses were surprised to find that she reacted aggressively to attempts to bath her and resisted their efforts to obtain a midstream specimen of urine. Attempts to make her feel at home by calling her Mary were met with an hostile reception, as did the approach of the auxiliary, who addressed her as Mrs. Jones. When the friend who had been on holiday with Miss Jones visited, she was distressed to find Miss Jones in tears and to hear the nurses describe her as an 'awkward old woman'.

1 What factors may have led to the failure of interaction?
2 What steps could be taken to retrieve the situation?

Author's Comments

Consider the following points (not necessarily inclusive):

1 Cultural variation between North and South of England as it affects:
  (a) ways in which people are addressed, eg, 'love' or by first name;
  (b) possible dialect difficulties, especially if patient has slight hearing loss, leading to lack of understanding;
  (c) may resent being addressed as 'Mrs' when single.
2 Age variation between patient and nurses
  (a) latter young, like those previously taught? Resentment of being ordered about;
  (b) patient may be a lot more intelligent than nurses who, because she is old may well 'talk down' to her;
  (c) resentment at 'young girls' helping with private and intimate tasks, such as elimination, washing.
3 In the geriatric ward, even though alert and intelligent, she may have resented comparison with those less able and confused (? element of fear that she may become like them).

All these facts may lead to aggression in an effort to maintain 'self-image'.

References and Further Reading

Blumer (1964) Society as Symbolic Interaction, In *Human Behaviour and Social Process* Rose A M (Ed) 1972 pp 179-192. Routledge and Kegan Paul, London.

King I M (1971) *Towards a Theory for Nursing.* J. Wiley and Sons, New York

This is a basic text which introduces King's model and discusses in detail its components. It also discusses a major interacting system, individuals, groups and society.

King I , (1981) *A Theory of Nursing.* J. Wiley and Sons, New York.

This contains some of the material from King (1971), but with further discussion. It also includes a goal-orientated nursing record.

Mead G H (1934) *Mind, Self and Society from the Standpoint of a Social Behaviourist,* University of Chicago Press

Rose A M (1980) A systematic summary of symbolic interaction theory. In *Conceptual Models for Nursing Practice,* Part II, Riehl J P & Roy C (Eds). Appleton-Century-Crofts, New York

This is an explanation of assumptions in social psychological theory to explain symbolic interaction based on the works of Mead, Gestalt, theorists and others. This text is a clear summary of the subject.

Roth I (1963) *Timetables: Structuring the Passage of Time in Hospital Treatment and Other Cares.* Bobbs Merrill Co., Indianapolis

Scott W R (1966) Professionals in bureaucracy; areas of conflict, In *Professionalisation,* ed. Vollner H H; 272-4, Prentice Hall, London

Singh A (1972) Personality needs of an English sample of student nurses. *Nursing Times* (occasional paper) **68** (12).

Timasheff N S (1966) *Sociological Theory: Its Nature and Growth.* (p4) Random House, New York

Thomas W I & Znancechi F (1927) *Primitive Behaviour: The Polish Peasant in Europe and America,* Denver Publications, New York.

CHAPTER SEVEN

BEHAVIOURAL MODELS

The behavioural models discussed here are based on the preposition that human beings are normally able to function in society by their own efforts. This activity may be variously described as 'meeting their own needs' (Henderson, 1964), carrying our 'activities of living' (Roper, 1976) or 'meeting their own self-care requirements' (Orem, 1980).

Such models owe much to the hierarchy of human needs (Figure 7.1), as analysed by Maslow (1970). This hierarchy starts at the bottom, with the needs essential to life and, as these are met, progresses up the pyramid until the ability of the individual to fulfil his potential is achieved.

Henderson stated that:

> 'The unique function of the nurse is to assist the individual, sick or well, in the performance of those activities contributing to health or its recovery (or to peaceful death) that he would perform unaided if he had the necessary strength, will or knowledge. And to do this in such a way as to help him gain independence as rapidly as possible.'

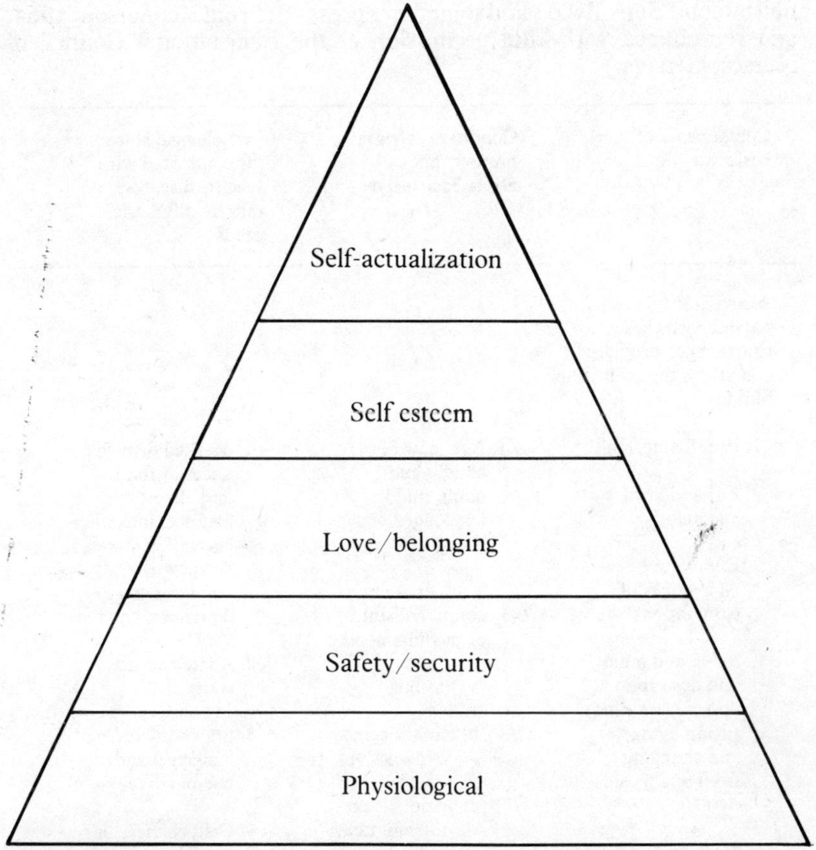

Figure 7.1 Hierarchy of human needs (From Maslow, *Activation and Personality*, 2nd Edn., with kind permission of Harper & Row, New York. 1970)

However, she acknowledges that, while nursing care may be derived from human needs, so do all welfare services. This means that the nurse is required to work as a member of a caring team, with some aspects of care being more adequately met by other members of the team.

Henderson listed the needs usually met by the nurse (Table 7.1).

Table 7.1 Needs of the patient met by the nurse, and how these are modified by conditions always and sometimes present. (From Henderson, 1964, and reproduced with kind permission of the International Council of Nurses, Geneva.)

Components of basic nursing	Conditions always present that affect basic needs	Pathological state (as contrasted with specific diseases) that modify basic needs
Assisting the patient with these functions or providing conditions that will enable him to:		
1. Breathe normally	1. Age: new born, child, youth, adult, middle-aged, aged and dying.	1. Marked disturbances of fluid and electrolyte balance, including starvation states, pernicious vomiting and diarrhoea
2. Eat and drink adequately	2. Temperament, emotional state or passing mood:	2. Acute oxygen want
3. Eliminate by all avenues of elimination	(a) 'normal'	3. Shock (including 'collapse' and haemorrhage)
4. Move and maintain desirable posture (walking, sitting, lying and changing from one to the other)	(b) euphoric and hyperactive	4. Disturbances of consciousness — fainting, coma, delirium
5. Sleep and rest	(c) anxious, fearful, agitated, or hysterical	5. Exposure to cold and heat causing markedly abnormal body temperatures
6. Select suitable clothing, dress and undress	(d) depressed and hypoactive	6. Acute febrile states (all causes)
7. Maintain body temperature within normal range by adjusting clothing and modifying the environment	3. Social or cultural status:	

Components of basic nursing	Conditions always present that affect basic needs	Pathological state (as contrasted with specific diseases) that modify basic needs
8. Keep the body clean and well groomed and protect the integument	a member of a family unit with friends and status, or a person relatively alone and/or maladjusted, destitute	7. A local injury, wound and/or infection
		8. A communicable condition
9. Avoid dangers in the environment and avoid injuring others.	4. Physical and intellectual capacity:	9. Pre-operative state.
	(a) normal weight	10. Post-operative state.
10. Communicate with others in expressing emotions, needs, fears, etc	(b) underweight	11. Immobilization from disease or prescribed as treatment
	(c) overweight	
11. Worship according to his faith	(d) normal mentality	12. Persistent or intractable pain
	(e) subnormal mentality	
12. Work at something that provides a sense of accomplishment	(f) gifted mentality	
13. Play, or participate in various forms of recreation	(g) normal sense of hearing, sight, equilibrium and touch	
14. Learn, discover or satisfy the curiosity that leads to 'normal' development and health	(h) loss of special sense	
	(i) normal motor power.	
	(j) loss of motor power	

While it is true that these basic needs exist regardless of the diagnostic category of the patient, nevertheless the disease process modifies them.

Roper (1976) elaborated a similar model to that of Henderson, although she described the patients' needs in terms of 'activities of living', that is the observable behaviours based on needs.

Twelve activities of living are specified:

1 Maintaining a safe environment
2 Communicating
3 Breathing
4 Eating and drinking
5 Eliminating
6 Personal cleansing and dressing
7 Controlling body temperatures
8 Mobilizing
9 Working and playing
10 Expressing sexuality
11 Sleeping
12 Dying.

Such activities are concerned with the person's whole life span from conception to death. Throughout life there is also a continuum of dependency, associated with age and health state, by which the individual moves in either direction.

These types of activity may be classified as 'preventing' (eg, handwashing), 'comforting' (eg, going to bed with a hot drink when feeling unwell) and 'seeking' (eg, looking for new knowledge and experiences). The result of these components is a model which can be displayed as shown in Figure 7.2

The patient's state on the continuum — totally dependent to totally independent — can be charted for each activity of living and care planned to either help move the line towards the independent end or, in the case of chronic illness or pending death, instigate nursing care which will support the patient in a dependent state (Figure 7.3).

Activities of living: preventing comforting seeking	Conception —— Life-span ——→ Death Totally dependent ←— Continuum —→ totally independent.
Maintaining a safe environment	
Communication	
Breathing	
Eating and drinking	
Eliminating	
Personal cleansing and dressing	
Controlling body temperature	
Mobilizing	
Working and playing	
Expressing sexuality	
Sleeping	
Dying	

Figure 7.2 Model of living (From Roper, Logan and Tierney 1980, *The Elements of Living*, reproduced by kind permission of Churchill Livingstone, Edinburgh)

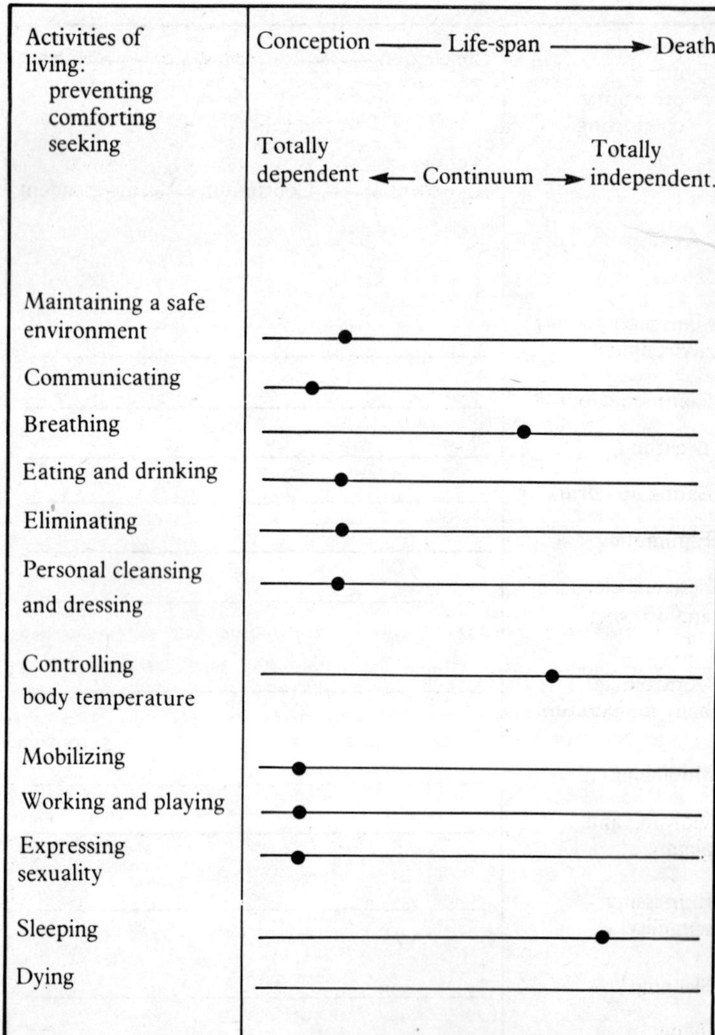

Figure 7.3 Model of living: a 60-year-old patient following a cerebral haemorrhage (From Roper, Logan & Tierney 1980, *The Elements of Living*, reproduced by kind permission of Churchill Livingstone, Edinburgh)

Orem (1980) first introduced her model of self-care in 1959 and has refined it since that date. The model is based on the statement that the individuals who benefit from nursing care are those who have self-care limitations, and that when self-care is not maintained, then illness, disease or death will result. She defined self-care requisites as universal, developmental and health-deviation self-care requisites.

Universal Self-Care Requisites

1 The maintenance of a sufficient intake of air.
2 The maintenance of a sufficient intake of water.
3 The maintenance of a sufficient intake of food.
4 The provision of care associated with elimination processes and excrement.
5 The maintenance of a balance between activity and rest.
6 The maintenance of a balance between solitude and social interaction.
7 The prevention of hazards to human life, human functioning and human well-being.
8 The promotion of human functioning and development within social groups in accord with human potential, known human limitations and the human desire to be normal. Normalcy is used in the sense of that which is essentially human and that which is in accord with the genetic and constitutional characteristics and the talents of individuals.

Developmental Self-Care Requisites

1 The bringing about and maintenance of living conditions that support life processes and promote the processes of development during various stages of life, with consideration given to each universal self-care requisite during:
(a) the intrauterine stages of life and the process of birth;
(b) the neonatal stage of life;

(c) infancy;
(d) the developmental stages of childhood and adolescence;
(e) the developmental stages of adulthood; and
(f) pregnancy either in adolescence or adulthood.

2 Provision of care either to prevent the occurrence of deleterious effects of conditions that can affect human development, or to mitigate or overcome these effects, such as:

(a) educational deprivation;
(b) problems of social adaptation;
(c) failures of healthy individuation;
(d) loss of relatives, friends and associates;
(e) loss of possessions or of occupational security;
(f) abrupt change of residence to an unfamiliar environment;
(g) status-associated problems;
(h) poor health or disability;
(i) oppressive living conditions; and
(j) terminal illness and impending death.

Health-Deviation Self-Care Requisites

1 Seeking and securing appropriate medical assistance in the event of exposure to specific physical or biological agents, or environmental conditions associated with human pathological events and states, or when there is evidence of genetic, physiological or psychological conditions known to produce or be associated with human pathology.
2 Being aware of and attending to the effects and results of pathological conditions and states.
3 Effectively carrying out medically prescribed diagnostic, therapeutic and rehabilitative measures directed to the prevention of specific types of pathology, to the pathology itself, to the regulation of human integrated functioning, to the correction of deformities or abnormalities, or to compensation for disabilities.

4 Being aware of and attending to, or regulating, the discomforting or deleterious effects of medical care measures performed or prescribed by the physician.
5 Modifying the self-concept (and self-image) in accepting oneself as being in a particular state of health and in need of specific forms of health care.
6 Learning to live with the effects of pathological conditions and states and the effects of medical diagnostic and treatment measures in a life-style that promotes continued personal development.

The Goal of Nursing

The goal of nursing is to help people meet their own self-care demands and, when that is not possible, assist in the adjustment to dependence. The nurse may also function by assisting relatives to help provide this care. Indeed, Orem (1980) identified five methods of action by the nurse:

1 Acting or doing for another.
2 Guiding another.
3 Supporting another physically or psychologically.
4 Providing an environment that promotes personal development
5 Teaching another.

Summary

All these models share a similar approach, that of identification of a deficit in the physiological, psychological or social functioning of the patient. They also therefore demonstrate a way in which the need for nursing interaction may be identified and, as a consequence, the way in which the effectiveness of nursing interaction may be measured.

Health Care Profile

Another model which has within it a method of measurement of

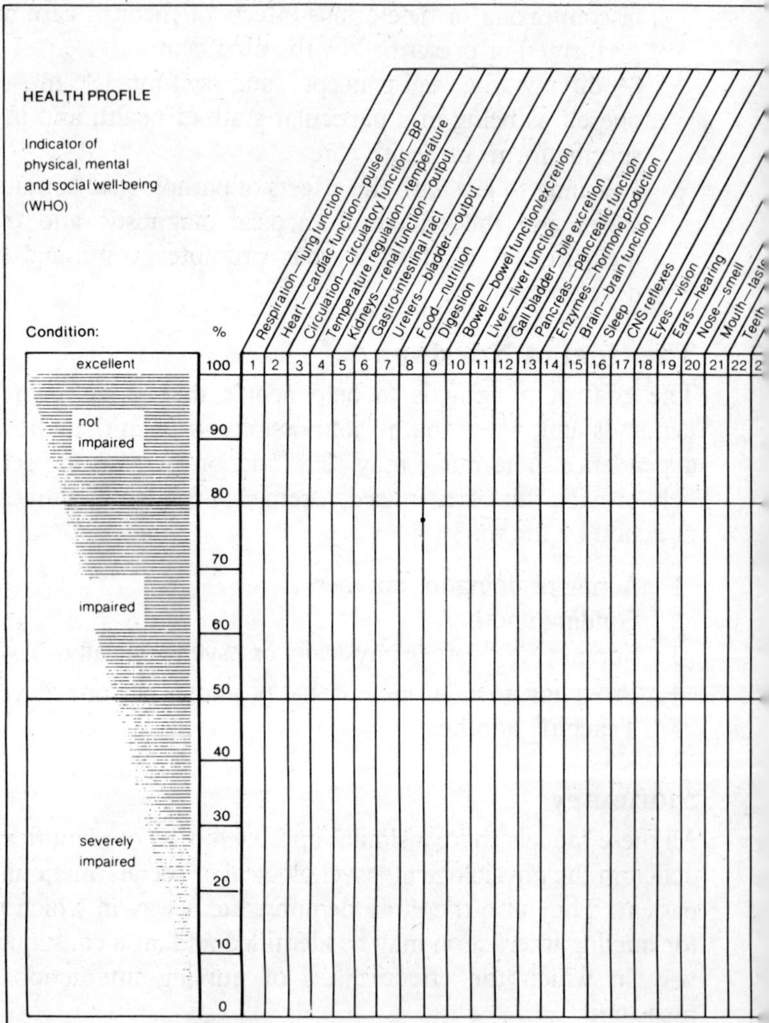

Figure 7.4 A health profile form (From Borsig 1979, *The health pr*
of *Nursing Times*, MacMillan Journals).

…obility / …eet/mobility / …pine—mobility

	Glands, endocrine, exocrine/function	Genitalia	Blood—reticulo-endothelial system	Environmental factors	Mental health	Family situation	Feelings of embarrassment	Pain	Fear	Depression	Development	Family/partner relationship	Sexuality	Friends	Social standing	Success	Role expectations	Financial security	Home/living conditions	Job—profession	Ability to work	Recreation	Sports—games	Holidays—vacation	Travel							
	31	32	33	34	35	36	37	38	39	40	41	42	43	44	45	46	47	48	49	50	51	52	53	54	55							
…th care																																

…by kind permission

change is the Health Care Profile developed in 1977 by Anna von Gottberg and Annemarie Borsig (1979). The core of this model is health and illness and the definition of health is that put forward by the World Health Organization: 'Health is a state of complete physical, mental and social wellbeing, and not merely the absence of illness or disease'. Such a statement is, of course, the ideal, and many persons will have some deviation from the complete state of well-being and yet not be classified ill in the usual sense (compare a person who is short-sighted and wears glasses). Because of this, the profile incorporates a scale 1-100 for 58 different physical, psychological and social states. A score of 80-100 is classified as 'health not impaired', 50-80 as 'impaired' and below 50 as 'severely impaired' (requires supervision, care, treatment and rehabilitation). Figures 7.4 and 7.5 demonstrate these points: Figure 7.4 is the Health Profile on which the patient's state is marked in the form of a graph, and Figure 7.5 indicates into which category the need for nursing intervention occurs.

One of the strengths of this type of recording of the patient's base-line condition is that subsequent recordings indicate movement in response to nursing intervention. Secondly, the involvement of the patient/client in the completion of this type of assessment will often demonstrate the different perception held by the person being assessed and the assessor.

Exercise

Using one of these models, demonstrate how you would assess the need for nursing care, the plan of nursing intervention and the way in which its effect could be measured for a 65-year-old man with rheumatoid arthritis who is being nursed at home by his 64-year-old wife.

Author's Comments

In the assessment, did you cover the physical, psychological and social state? Consider the possible assessment that would have been

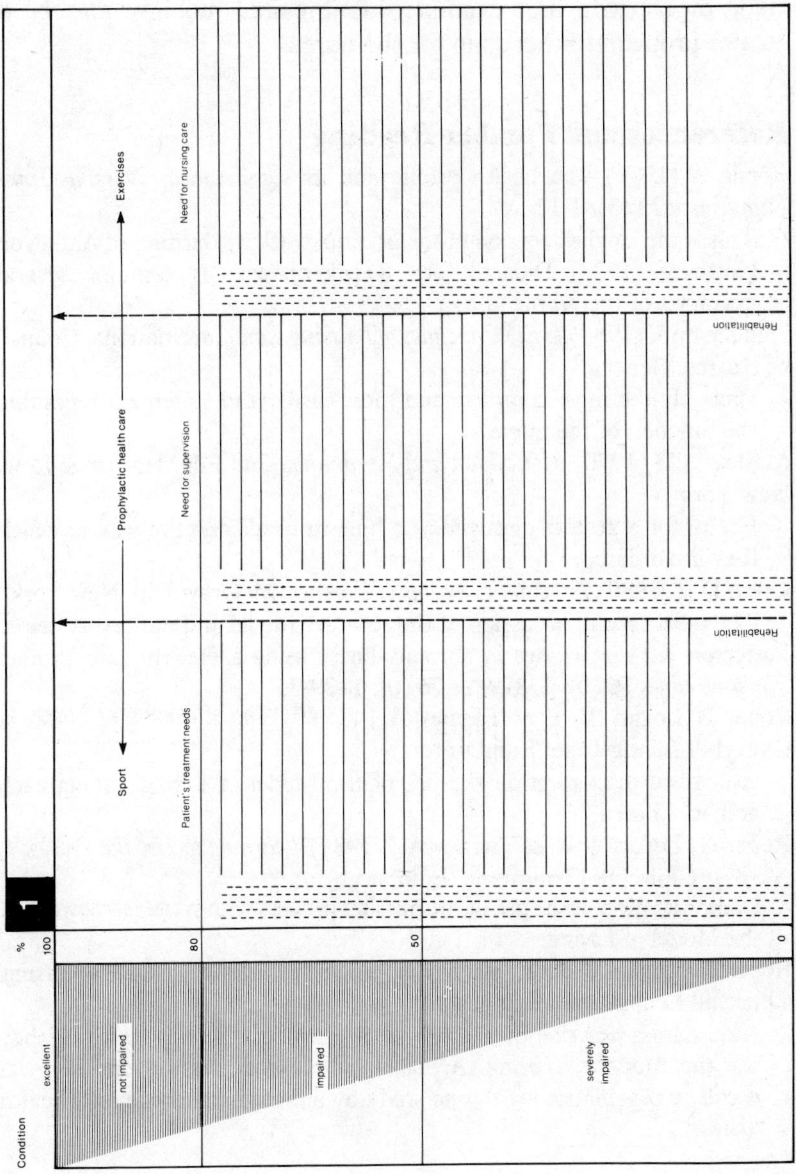

Figure 7.5 The categorization of a patient's needs following completion of health profile (From Borsig 1979, *The health profile*, reproduced by kind permission of *Nursing Times*, MacMillan Journals)

made by his wife. For example, his impaired mobility may be a greater problem for her than for the nurse.

References and Further Reading

Börsig A (1979) The health profile and its significance. *Nursing Times Supplement* **75** (3): 1-12

This is the English version of the original work in German of Anna von Gottberg (1977) Didactik der Krankenpflege. It contains several examples of the profile in use.

Henderson V (1964) *Basic Principles of Nursing Care*, International Council of Nurses, Geneva

Probably the most complete and most easily read statement regarding the function of the nurse.

Maslow A H (1970) *Motivation and Personality*, 2nd Edn. Harper & Row, New York

Useful for a greater discussion on human needs and the way in which they are ordered.

Orem D E (1980) *Nursing: Concepts of Practice.* McGraw Hill, New York

The most recent discussion of the self-care model and nursing systems.

Patterson K (1980) Care in chronic illness using a Health Care Profile. *Nursing Times* **76** (0): 1387-9 & **76** (0): 1429-35

Roper N Logan W W & Tierney A J (1980) *The Elements of Nursing.* Churchill Livingstone, Edinburgh

A detailed discussion on the use of the Model of Living, taking each activity in turn.

Roper N, Logan W W & Tierney A J (1981) *Learning to Use the Process of Nursing.* Churchill-Livingstone, Edinburgh

Demonstration of the use of the nursing process within the framework of the Model of Living.

Roper N, Logan W W & Tierney A J (1983) *Using a Model for Nursing.* Churchill Livingstone, Edinburgh.

Nine nurses describe by the use of case studies, the way in which they use the Model of Living. Areas of care include medical and surgical wards, a psychiatric ward, one study by a midwife and one by a health visitor

PART III

DELIVERY OF CARE

CHAPTER EIGHT

THE NURSING PROCESS

At various points during the preceding chapters, reference has been made to the need to assess the patient's requirements for patient care, to the way in which such care may be planned, and whether or not goals set are achieved. This is the logical approach to any activity:

1	*Assessment:*	What needs to be done?
2	*Plan:*	How may the above needs be met? Are there alternative methods? Which methods are the best? Goals set in order of priority.
3	*Action:*	Record of steps taken in line with the plan.
4	*Evaluation:*	Have the goals been met? Was the action appropriate? Are new goals required?

Assessment

In order to plan individualized nursing care, it is necessary to identify the patient's needs or problems. To do this, the information may be gained directly from the patient, or if the patient is incapable of communicating for any reason (eg, too young, confused, unconscious), relatives or friends may provide the data. In addition, material may be available from the doctor's case notes. Certain physical signs, such as temperature level, pulse rate and blood pressure, may be obtained by measurement or examination.

To obtain this information, many institutions use a standardized questionnaire, with some questions merely requiring a (✓), while others may require elaboration and explanation. The information may be classified into:

1 Personal indentification, eg, name, address, age, marital status, etc.
2 Social — relating to housing, occupation, relatives.
3 Physical — current health and past medical history.
4 Normal activities — sleep, eating habits, elimination.
5 Senses — hearing, vision, etc.
6 Psychological — patient's emotional response to admission and illness.

When making the assessment of the patient, it is important that the nurse endeavours to perceive the situation as it is seen by the patient and/or his relatives, as well as noting the objective measures or the view of the situation as seen by herself and/or a medical colleague. Some examples of this apparently subjective view are:

A patient who all his life may have had defective vision which has been corrected by glasses will be unlikely to consider this 'a problem', while the fact that he has not had his bowels opened in the past 24 hours may seem highly important. Patients who are admitted following an accident are frequently more concerned with the fact that they are expected at work or have tickets for the theatre than they are with injuries. These examples indicate the importance that people attach to their social roles and the fact that as long as they are able to fulfil them they do not consider themselves 'ill'.

This social aspect of the patient's life must be taken into account in all stages of care and, in particular, when goals are being set related to discharge.

Figures 8.1 and 8.2 show two examples of assessment forms: the patient's assessment form and the patient's profile.

Care Plan

Once the assessment of needs has been made, the next step is to decide how these needs may be met and whether there is any priority in action required. This needs consideration of alternative methods of care and, following the decision as to the most appropriate method, the plan of care can then be written. This plan may be demonstrated as a problem-solving activity as shown in Figure 8.3.

It is important that the goals, or sub-goals, set are realistic so that progress can be seen and that they are understood and agreed by the patient and, in some cases, the relatives, as well as by the nursing staff. Cooperation by all is vital and often great misery is caused by patients not understanding the reason behind nursing action.

Evaluation

In Figure 8.3 there is a column labelled 'nursing action', and a column labelled 'result'. This record of the outcome of nursing interaction is vital. In the example shown in Figure 8.3, it might read level with goal 1:

'Sixth day was able to walk to the toilet with help'.

This would indicate that the strategy of gradually moving the chair further away from the bed has succeeded in its purpose.

Following this evaluation, goal 2 can be set, and so on. Any failure

NURSING ADMISSION SHEET
*Record Number ______
PATIENT LABEL
*Name ______
*Address ______

*Date of birth ______ *Age ______
*Date of admission ______ *Time ______
*Type: Emergency Waiting List
*Transfer from ______
*Marital status ______ *Religion ______
*Next of kin (name) ______
*Relationship to patient ______
*Address ______

*Tel. no(s). ______

Speech difficulty/language barrier ______

CARE AT HOME Details/Names
Community Nurse ______

Social Worker ______

Social Services (specify) ______

*GP (name) ______
*Address ______

*Consultant ______
*House Officer ______
*Diagnosis ______

*Operations on present admission/date performed: ______

*Past medical history/operations ______

*Allergies ______

*History of present complaint ______

*Other current health problems ______

*What patient says is the reason for admission ______

NURSING REMINDERS ______

SOCIAL HISTORY Occupation ______
Children ______
Other dependents ______
HOUSING (house, flat — which floor, stairs, lives alone, shares, bathroom/toilet) ______

Other problems at home? ______

Visiting problems? Yes No
If Yes, describe ______
DISCHARGE PLANNING — Please tick those required, add date when ordered or done

	Needed	Date ordered
Social Services (specify) ______	______	______
Community Nurse	______	______
*TTA's and Teaching	______	______
*Out-patient's appt.	______	______
*Transport	______	______
*Relatives informed	______	______

Figure 8.1 A patient assessment form

DAILY LIVING

DIET
*Special ______
Food or drink dislikes ______
Appetite: Good Poor
Remarks ______

SLEEP How many hours usually? ______
Sedation ______
Other comments ______

ELIMINATION
BOWELS Any problems: Yes No
If Yes, describe ______
How often are bowels opened? ______
Any medication? ______
URINARY No problems Incontinence
Nocturia Dysuria
Frequency Urgency
Remarks ______

FEMALE PATIENTS — MENSTRUATION
Regular Irregular
Amenorrhoea Dysmenorrhoea
Post-menopausal Taking the pill
Next period due ______
Will need: ST's Tampons
Remarks ______

HEARING Right: Good Poor Deaf
Left: Good Poor Deaf
Hearing Aid? Yes No
Remarks ______

VISION Right: Good Poor Blind
Left: Good Poor Blind
Glasses Contact Lenses
Remarks ______

PROSTHESES/APPLIANCE/AIDS
Type(s) ______
Any help needed? No Yes ______

MOBILITY Fully mobile? Yes No
If No, needs help with:
Walking Standing Dressing
Washing Bathing Feeding
In/out of bed In/out of chair
Other (describe) ______

ORAL
Any problems with mouth or teeth?
Yes No
If Yes, Decribe ______
Wears dentures?
No Yes: Upper Lower
Any problems with dentures? ______
Any crowns? ______

SMOKING HABITS Non-smoker
Smokes: pipe cigars cigarettes

NURSE'S OBSERVATIONS

*ATTITUDE
Anxious Withdrawn Distressed
Remarks (If particular problem please try and state reason, e.g. anxious about operation/or being in hospital, etc.) ______

GENERAL APPEARANCE
Normal Obese
Dehydrated Thin
Acutely ill Emaciated
Remarks ______

SKIN
Satisfactory Broken areas
Dehydrated Rash
Oedematous Jaundiced
Describe ______

LEVEL OF CONSCIOUSNESS
Orientated Semi-conscious
Confused Unconscious
Remarks ______

NORTON SCORE: ______

Information obtained: From By Level of training/position Date Time

Figure 8.1 A patient assessment form

PATIENT PROFILE		
Addressograph	**Social**	**Additional Information**
Medical cert. Required/given Employment cert. Required/given	Occupation Marital status Dependents (including pets) Lives alone Yes/No Type of accommodation	
Valuables		
Next of kin Person to contact if different	Problems caused by hospitalization Financial	
Community Care G.P. DN/HV Social worker Social services Religious minister.	Hobbies/interests.	

Figure 8.2 A patient profile

PATIENT PROFILE		
Addressograph		**Sleep Pattern** **Sedation**
Reason for admission/diagnosis	Attitude	**Elimination** Bowel Aperient Urinary
Patient/family reason for admission	Level of consciousness/awareness	**Hygiene** Condition of skin Condition of mouth Dentures
Past medical history	Mobility	**Nutrition** State Likes/dislikes Appetite Special diet Problems
Additional health problems	Sensory Hearing Aid Vision Loss of Sensation Speech/Language	Last menstrual period Post menopausal Problems
Medication on admission Disposal:		

Figure 8.2 cont.

Problem	Goal or Subgoal	Nursing Action	Result
Difficulty in walking	1. To be able to walk to toilet with help in 7 days	1. Assist patient to walk to chair and back at least three times daily. Daily move chair further away from bed.	
	2. To be able to walk to the toilet unaided prior to discharge.	2. Walk with patient to toilet, but not offering support unless in danger of falling.	

Figure 8.3 Part of a patient care plan

to reach the goal means either that the aim was unrealistic, or that the method to achieve that goal was inappropriate. Either way, a fresh assessment of that specific part of the patient's care is required and a new plan evolved.

Framework of Care

Any of the theories or models already mentioned may be used as a framework for the nursing process. For example 'difficulty in walking' can be shown under the following headings where in each case, there is recognition that normally an individual is able to walk about unaided and therefore nursing care must be focused on returning the individual to that condition, if at all possible:

V. Henderson
Patient's need to move and maintain desirable posture.

N. Roper
Activity of living — mobilizing.

D. Orem
Self-care requisite, the maintenance of a balance between activity and rest.

Exercise

Obtain a set of nursing process documents from your own institution. Consider the following questions:

1 On what basis are they constructed, eg, are they problem-orientated, or otherwise?
2 Is there evidence of a framework of a nursing model?
3 Is it possible to see clearly the goals set for the outcome of nursing activity?

If the answer to question 2 is 'Yes', see if you can use the same documents with a different model.

If the answer to question 2 is 'No', try to design a form using one of the models described in this book.

Author's Comments

The use of a nursing model helps ensure that all aspects of normal living are considered when assessing the patient, and also makes goal setting more precise.

References and Further Reading

Henderson V (1964) *Basic Principles of Nursing Care.* International Council of Nurses, Geneva

Orem D E (1980) *Nursing: Concepts of Practice.* McGraw Hill, New York

Roper N Logan W W & Tierney A J (1981) *Learning to Use the Process of Nursing.* Churchill Livingstone, Edinburgh

Nursing Process

In addition to the above, the following texts deal in detail with the use of the nursing process.

Hunt J M & Marks-Maran D J (1980) *Nursing Care Plans.* H.M. & M Publishers, Aylesbury

Mariner A (1975) *The Nursing Process. A Scientific Approach to Nursing Care.* C.V. Mosby, St. Louis

McFarlane J & Castledine G (1982) *A Guide to the Practice of Nursing Using the Nursing Process.* C. V. Mosby & Co., London

CHAPTER NINE

THEORY RELATED TO THE NURSE

Nurses' Needs

One of the advantages of using a 'needs' model as a framework for care is that the concept can apply to relatives and the carers (doctors, nurses, etc) just as readily as it can to patients.

Indeed, while there is constant emphasis placed on the fact that the patient or client must be considered on an individual basis and not just seen as a member of a diagnostic or need category, it is rare for this consideration to be given to those giving the care.

Nevertheless, nurses are human and do have individual needs, some of which they seek to fulfil by the activity of caring for others. Many studies have been made as to why people wish to nurse and to why some become 'wasted' (MacGuire, 1966). Reasons given by neophytes for entering nursing are usually those of wishing to work with people, or statements indicating a desire to help those less fortunate than themselves. Some will add to such reasons the desire to learn more about disease and its treatment, others may indicate a desire to develop technical skills. A few may admit to wanting a worthwhile career and, although it is unlikely to be openly admitted, some may be seeking an avenue for social mobility. These then are the goals or needs of the nurse but, as discussed, the patient also has goals and needs. The prime need of the patient is the return to health and normal functioning, but there may be many subsidiary needs to be met along the path. The goals of the nurse and the patient may be the same, may complement each other, or may be in conflict. This situation has been developed in the interaction model by King (1971).

Social anthropologists and sociologists such as Malinowski (1922) and Homans (1961) have developed a theory of 'social-exchange' to explain some of the ways individuals interact with one another. Cynics argue that little is done in the world from purely altruistic motives, but that in every activity there is a reward. Certainly it is necessary to look for a reward to explain why individuals not only take up, but continue in the activity of nursing; an occupation which demands unsocial hours, hard physical work, unpleasant sights and sounds, contact with people in their least attractive moments, emotional tension, grief and death. What keeps nurses at their job and explains why many of them 'would not do anything else?' Not all stay, however, and those who leave express varying degrees of disenchantment and frustration either with the task, the way it is organized, or with other apparently less tangible factors.

The position of health care within the United Kingdom is such that it has frequently been considered 'free' because payment does not have to be made at the point of delivery, although this perception is rapidly changing. Indeed, since levels of pay for the nursing profession have been increased, some patients feel that the nurse is caring for them not because she has a vocation, but because she is paid to do a job. Other patients feel, however, that the care they receive is greater than that which is paid for either by their contributions or by the salary that the nurse receives. In the latter case, there is an interesting relationship. The nurse may be seen to be the giver of a gift, that of her care, and the patient the receiver without the normal provision for the return of gifts, indeed individual gifts from patients to nurses are officially frowned on. In fact, the return of a gift, as occurs with birthday or Christmas presents, demands a degree of equality of relationship between the giver and the receiver which, during the time that the individual is receiving nursing care, does not exist. Although the patient may only be in a state of temporary dependence, in the case of the chronic sick, handicapped or dying, the dependence may be permanent so here repayment for nursing may be considered to be impossible.

It is this inequality of relationship that places nursing in the category of occupations which are considered vocational by the general public and which gives nursing much of its status. An effort to restore the balance is frequently made by patients by the gift of gratitude and Simmel describes this as the 'supplement' which seeks to restore the imbalance (Wolfe, 1964).

However, if the reasons why individuals take up nursing are noted, it may be that they are repaid in other ways. For example, the dependence of the patient may satisfy a nurse's psychological needs. Nurses themselves tend to indicate that this is the situation and, if not prevented, they may increase or prolong the patient's dependency. It is the complaint of many patients in hospital that they are not allowed to carry out normal physical activities that are well within their competence, and that by both conversation and care they are reduced to the level of children.

Titmuss (1970) calls this activity 'creative altruism', creative in the sense that the self is realized with the help of others. He, in discussing blood-donors, says that giving blood 'allows the biological need to help to express itself'. Tönnies (1887) sees such activity more cynically, saying 'Do, ut, des', 'What I do for you, I do only as a means to effect your simultaneous, previous or later service for me . . . To get something from you is my end, my service is thereto which I contribute unwillingly'. Maybe this sort of statement throws light on the fact that the care of some classes of patients is seen as less prestigious in the eyes of society, which tends to classify the worth of individuals in relation to the contribution they are able to make to society. It is not difficult to see that the stigma of dependency rests most heavily on the old, the chronically sick, the mentally handicapped and those who are unlikely to recover and become givers to society. This stigmatization may also become attached to those who care for such people and may account for the fact that nurses who consider their calling a true vocation (eg members of religious orders) particularly concentrate on these groups. Pinker (1971) has described this situation, where the individual is unlikely to be able to repay, as one where the person is perpetually subject to a 'compassion gap'. Furthermore, he points out that the relationship between the giver and the receiver is always inherently an unstable and unequal one and that though gratitude may be used to help restore the balance, because a gift is given first, it may be given with a sense of coercion. Money is the commodity which produces instant equivalence, and even the interest paid on money borrowed shows that the lack of equivalence is only temporary. Gratitude is not seen in this light and it is generally agreed that is more blessed to give than receive.

The model of scales shown in Figure 9.1 demonstrates the importance of the interaction between the nurse and patient and the way in which nurses' needs may be met by the care they are required to give to the patient.

This interaction, as a form of social-exchange, illustrates the goals and needs of both the patient and the nurse. A plus sign indicates attributes or skills available and a minus sign indicates deficiencies that have to be made up if the integrity of the individual is to be maintained and his needs met.

If the plus and minus signs in Figure 9.1 are added up this may indicate that there is an imbalance, with the nurse in credit and the patient remaining in debt. However, there is no indication as to the strength or depth of any of these factors, ie, if 'weighting' could be carried out, the result might be different. Also the nurse may receive other rewards from society, such as social esteem and/or social

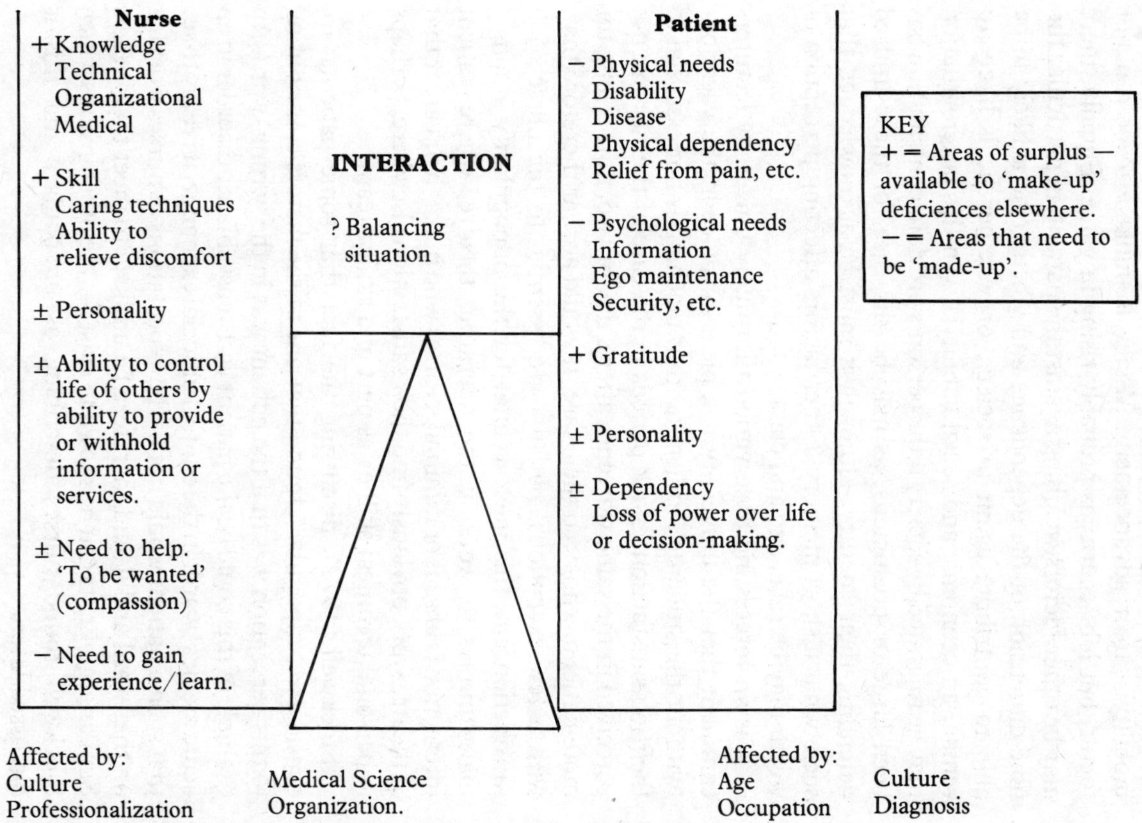

Figure 9.1 A model of the nurse/patient interaction process and the maintenance of equilibrium

mobility, career advancement. Money is unlikely to be a major factor, but job security is probably rising in value. Equally, there may be other factors weighing against the patient, in particular the time dimension of the dependency and whether he is likely to be able to contribute again to society, or whether he is likely to remain an economic and social liability. Even this latter situation may be tolerated by society if the person's previous contribution has been large or prestigious, as may be the case for those injured defending their country, although it must be acknowledged that society has a short memory. Other factors affecting perception of worth may be race, age and class.

It is an interesting observation that many university lecturers comment that the university is a pleasant place in the vacations 'without the students', indicating that teaching is not essential to their job satisfaction. Slack periods in the care of the sick are not perceived in the same way and, after a day or two, nurses long for more patients who need their care. It would appear therefore that, with a few exceptions, patients are essential to the nurse's job satisfaction and this may account for the unpopularity amongst many nurses to work in the operating theatre, where patient interaction is absent or minimal. Nurses who make their career that of theatre work obviously find their satisfaction elsewhere, perhaps in personal technical skill or as part of a skilled team.

Stockwell (1972), discussing the fact that some patients are considered 'unpopular', found that one of the factors contributing to this perception was that the patient was in the 'wrong' ward. An example of this could be the patient with a psychiatric disorder in an acute medical ward. In the context of social exchange, it is easy to see that such a patient would not fit the expectations of nurses working on that ward and would therefore be unlikely to meet their needs. Similar arguments can be shown to exist for the other groups which Stockwell found nurses describing as unpopular, and this is discussed later.

Summary

To summarize at this point, the social exchange theory may help explain the way both patients and nurses are able to satisfy their physical and psychosocial needs. Obviously, any specific interaction situation may terminate with a debt on one side or another. However, due to the multiplicity of interaction situations that will occur for each of the participants, these debts may ultimately be cancelled out as the interaction incidents are summated. Pinker (1971) asserts that 'Dependencies of a stigmatizing or humiliating nature are most likely to be avoided when the individual receives aid of a partial nature from a number of providers'. Litwak (1965), discussing aid given to families, also states 'Where the giver is never in the position to provide the entire service then he is not in a position to ask for complete subservience'. These observations are important when the organization of care is considered. It may be that the multiplicity of contacts which modern health care demands is not as dysfunctional, as is commonly believed, but that they assist in lessening the stigma on behalf of the patient. Menzies (1960) has shown that the ability to turn from one patient to the care of another is of value in the relief of stress and anxiety felt by nurses.

This discussion however should not be used to support the idea that task-orientated nursing is the best way of organizing patient care. Rather, efforts must be made to ensure that any nurse in a situation which either does not meet her needs, and/or is stressful, is given other areas of satisfaction and has adequate support from peers and supervisors in the stressful situation. Task-orientated care inhibits the face-to-face interaction needed if interaction in the terms of this model is to take place.

Equally, if nurse teaching and patient care is focused on a medical model — that is the patient is seen as a disease with symptoms rather than as a patient with needs — this will result in an imbalance on both sides of the scale. The nurse will be frustrated in meeting her need to 'care' and the patient may feel depersonalized and lack ego security. To maintain the balance, therefore, and to make up for frustration in one area, nurses may turn to other facets of the exchange process. For example, they may exhibit excessive power in their relationships with patients and relatives, or demand more money from society to reassure them that their position is important. If forced to think in terms of the medical model, they may feel that technical skills are the most rewarding and that cure is more vital than care. Others may react to the frustration of their needs by leaving the profession in order to find fulfilment elsewhere.

Meanwhile, the patient in an effort to maintain his self-regard may react by non-cooperation, either aggressively or in an apathetic manner.

Nurses' and Patients' Rights and Duties

What is meant by 'right' and 'duty'? The words 'responsibility' and 'duty' mean very similar things, as shown in Roget's Thesaurus. Benn and Peters (1959) argue that a right and a duty are different names for the same normative relation (ie, situation based on rules), varying according to the position from which the situation is regarded. In other words, one person's rights become another person's duties. Rights may also imply duties in another sense in that the enjoyment by an individual of specific rights is usually conditional on the performance by that individual of specific duties. In this case, the association of rights and duties is not a logical relationship but a moral one.

'We demand our rights' is a phrase heard chanted daily by one or another group of people. Everywhere there are movements with titles claiming specific rights for particular groups of people, such as women's rights, the rights of the unborn child. In recent years, most countries have introduced legislation to protect the rights of members of their society (an example in the United Kingdom is the Employment Protection Act), yet rarely in any of these activities is 'duty' mentioned.

What are the rights and responsibilities attributable to nurses and patients in their interaction with one another?

Once again the social exchange model may be useful to demonstrate the fact that if one side of a coin depicts a right, the other side brings a responsibility.

In recent years there has been a great deal of discussion on the 'rights' that patients have once they have assumed the patient role. The American Hospital Association produced 'A Patients' Bill of Rights' in 1972: 'with the expectation that observance of these rights will contribute to more effective patient care and greater satisfaction for the patient, his physician and the hospital organization'. This Bill does not include nursing care within its jurisdiction, but has been adapted by nurses in the USA.

1 The patient has the right to considerate and respectful care.
2 The patient has the right to obtain from his physician his diagnosis, treatment and prognosis in simple terms. He has the right to know, by name, the physician responsible for his care.
3 The patient has the right to know the details of a treatment or procedure before he gives his consent.
4 The patient has the right to refuse treatment and be informed of the medical consequences.
5 The patient has the right to privacy concerning his own medical care. Case discussion, consultation, examination and treatment are confidential.
6 The patient has the right to expect that all communications and records pertaining to his care should be treated as confidential.
7 The patient has the right to expect that a hospital will make a reasonable response to the patient's request for services available in the hospital. Transfer to another facility must be explained and deemed necessary.
8 The patient has the right to know if his hospital works with other health care and educational institutions, in so far as his care is concerned.
9 The patient has the right to refuse to participate in human experimentation research projects.

10 The patient has the right to know the medical services available to him upon his discharge from the hospital.
11 The patient has the right to examine and receive an explanation of his bill, regardless how the bill will be paid.
12 The patient has the right to know the hospital rules and regulations which concern him.

(Adapted from the Patient's Bill of Rights presented by the American Hospital Association).

In discussing the role of the patient, Talcott Parsons (1966) argued that the patient only has the right to be called 'sick' and therefore excused other roles and duties if he fulfils his responsibilities and seeks competent help, demonstrating both the desire and will to get better by following advice given.

Many nurses would add to this by asserting that the patient has a responsibility to allow them to care for them, dependence of the patient therefore satisfying one of their psychological needs. As discussed, to give physical care may thus be regarded by the nurse far less as a duty than a right. The nurse may also feel that the patient has a duty to cooperate and be grateful for this care.

Stockwell (1972) said that nurses liked patients who:

1 Were able to communicate readily with nurses.
2 Knew the nurses' names.
3 Were able to joke and laugh with the nurses.
4 Cooperated in being helped to get well and expressed determination to do so.

The nurses saw these responses from the patient as their right.

In return, they were prepared to reward such patients in the form of:

1 More time.
2 Personalized interaction.
3 Willingness to accept gifts and favours.
4 Allowing lapses in keeping the rules.

Patients, in turn, felt that they had the right to receive:

1 Skilled care; 'a nurse you can depend on'.
2 Attention to 'trivial matters'.
3 More information.
4 More opportunity to voice worries and needs.

These expectations are demonstrated in Table 9.2

Table 9.2 Expectation of Nurses' rights and patients' duties

Nurses' rights	Patients' duties
Cooperation	Cooperation
Gratitude	Recognition of nurse as individual
Recognition	Openness of communication
Happy environment	Cheerfulness.

The Code for Nurses (ethical concepts applied to nursing) adopted by the International Council of Nurses Council of National Representatives in Mexico City in May 1973, denotes four main areas of responsibility for the nurse:

To promote health.
To prevent illness.
To restore health.
To alleviate suffering.

Continuing the principle of one man's rights being another man's duties, we get the picture as shown in Table 9.3, with a complex social exchange between nurses and patients, each with their expectations of their 'rights', obligations and duties (Figure 9.2).

NURSE		PATIENT	
RIGHTS	RESPONSIBILITIES	RIGHTS	RESPONSIBILITIES
To have appropriate experience (especially learners)	To give: Skilled care	To receive: Skilled nursing care	To cooperate in treatment
			To conform to routine
To be recognised as individual	Individualized care	Individual recognition	To be grateful
To receive reward for work	Information	Information	
Status) ? from patient Gratitude) relatives Money) society			
To have happy patients	Emotional support	Ability to voice worries	To be cheerful

Figure 9.2 Rights and responsibilities of the Nurse and Patient

Table 9.3 Expectations of the Nurses' duties and the patients' rights

Nurses' duties	Patients' rights
To promote health	Health
To prevent illness	or
To restore health	peaceful
To alleviate suffering	death

Inevitably, such a pattern of expectations may be the source of conflict when nurses see as their 'right' some things that patients do not regard as a duty to them, and vica versa. Such a situation may produce patient complaints and/or poor staff morale and wastage.

As discussed, the use of the nursing process may help prevent this conflict. If the patient has a right to know about his condition and treatment, and this is one of the 'rights' patients demand, then the patient must be involved in goal-setting. Such openness and freedom of communication between nurse and patient will enable each to understand the other and appreciate each other's needs, goals and expectation. With such understanding, the granting of 'rights' and the assumptions of 'responsibilities' is more likely to occur than when the patient is seen purely as a receiver and the nurse the giver.

Patient cooperation in goal-setting requires nursing assessment, care planning and evaluation to be carried out in a systematic way, with appropriate consideration given to the patient's perception of his needs as well as to those that are objectively quantifiable. Equally, the patient's perception of treatment, care and progress must be given due weight.

Nurses claim that they enjoy interacting with the patient. It should be a short step to turn this often transitory interaction into a relationship which produces satisfaction on both sides; a true 'social-exchange'.

Exercise

Honestly list the factors in nursing that are important to you. Then answer the following questions:

1 How may my 'needs' be best met in nursing?
2 Is there any specific branch of nursing that will be more appropriate than another?
3 What must I be prepared to 'give' in order to receive what I need?
4 What are my main strengths and abilities?

Author's Comments

This assessment of your own needs and abilities can be used to assist you in planning the rest of your career.

If you have difficulty in assessing yourself, ask help from a colleague or tutor.

References and Further Reading

American Hospital Association (1972) *A Patient's Bill of Rights.* American Hospital Association, New York

Benn S I & Peters R S (1959) *Social Principles and the Democratic State.* Allen and Unwin, London

This book is a philosophical text.

Homans G C (1961) *Social Behaviour, Its Elementary Forms.* Harcourt, Brace and World, New York

Contains basic discussion on aspects of social exchange and requires a basis of sociological knowledge.

International Council of Nurses (1973) *Code for Nurses.* ICN, Geneva An ethical code.

King I M (1971) *Toward a Theory of Nursing.* J. Wiley and Sons, Chichester

Already discussed in chapter on Interaction Theory

Levi-Strauss C (1969) *The Elementary Structures of Kinship.* Beacon Press, Boston

Contains basic discussion on aspects of social exchange and requires a basis of sociological knowledge.

Litwak E (1965) Extended kin relations in a democratic society. In *Social Structure and the Family: Generational Relations*, Shanas E & Steib G (Eds), 303-04. Prentice Hall, London

See Levi-Strauss (1969) for comments.

Malinowski B (1922) *Argonauts of the Western Pacific.* Routledge and Kegan Paul, New York

See Levi-Strauss (1969) for comments

Mauss M (1925) *The Gift.* Translation (1950) Cunnison I. Free Press, New York

See Levi-Strauss (1969) for comments

Menzies I E P (1960) A case-study in the functioning of social systems as a defence against anxiety. *Human Relationships* **60**: 95-121 4

An account of the steps taken by nurses to reduce stress.

Parsons T (1966) On becoming a patient. In *A Sociological Framework for Patient Care.* Folta J R & Deck E S (Eds) J Wiley and Sons, Chichester

A sociological discussion on the way in which a person adopts the patient role

Pinker R (1971) *Social Theory and Social Policy.* Heinemann, London

Contains basic discussion on aspects of social exchange and requires a basis of sociological knowledge

Stockwell F (1972) *The Unpopular Patient.* Royal College of Nursing, London

An account of research conducted to find out why some patients are classified as 'unpopular'.

Titmuss R (1970) *The Gift Relationship.* Allen and Unwin, London

Contains basic discussion on aspects of social exchange and requires a basis of sociological knowledge

Tonnies F (1887) *Community and Associations.* Translation (1955) Loomis P, Routledge and Kegan Paul, London

See Titmuss (1970) for comments

Wolfe K H (ed) (1964) *The Sociology of George Simmel.* Free Press, London

See Titmuss (1970) for comments.

CHAPTER TEN

PERCEPTIONS OF CARE

Discussion throughout the previous chapter has been concerned with the way nursing may be perceived and the effect that this perception may have on the delivery of care.

The practice of nursing varies not only according to the model or theory which is put into operation, and the process by which patient need is assessed, care planned, implemented and assessed, but also as a result of the basic beliefs and attitudes of the nurse.

Patient/client and nurse do not exist in a vacuum, but are subjected to influences from the environment, to sociocultural and family pressures and to organizational goals.

Fundamental to the pressures are the beliefs held by all the participants of the intrinsic value of the individual, and the individual's right to life and/or death. Such beliefs do not imply that all people are the same, indeed quite the contrary. Instead, nursing is usually acknowledged to be founded on the belief that an individual is both ideosyncratic and of intrinsic worth. That is, while acknowledging that each person is different and has a different contribution to make to society, some apparently are more valued than others. Nevertheless, each person, because he/she is a unique living creature, is worthy of equal care and attention.

Such a statement is of great importance and almost inevitably produces a degree of tension. Is it possible to regard the down-and-out meths drinker as worthy of equal care as the mother supporting five children, or the research scientist pioneering new fields of treatment? If not, then feet are already on the slippery slope which may lead ultimately to a decision such as that taken in Nazi Germany that only those of Aryan blood were fit to inherit the earth.

Such recognition of the intrinsic worth of an individual does not of course demand that they should be left in the state in which they are found. Therefore a second belief which nurses must hold is that nursing is an activity which 'makes a difference' to the individual receiving care. This difference may be seen in the meeting of needs that the patient is either no longer able to meet himself, or did not have the knowledge or insight to know were unfulfilled; needs met in order to assist the patient to recovery, maintain his present position, or to achieve a peaceful death. As discussed these needs may be expressed in a variety of ways, using different terminology, but the implications for action are the same. However, nursing may also be seen as 'a mechanism for change' not only as to the state of the patient, but also in a wider context. Nurses occupy a unique position in that they are able to influence patients; their own attitude to the individual may well affect his to other people. As a large group of people, they are also in a position to act as a pressure group in both local and national politics on vital issues affecting the intrinsic worth of the individual (an example of this was seen when nurses reacted to a proposed bill introduced in the House of Lords on Euthanasia).

Indeed, in the issues of life and death, the nurse needs to be very sure of her own beliefs so that she can help others. In western culture, death is still regarded as taboo in normal conversation. Indeed poets seem to be the only people who apparently feel comfortable in writing about death (see the large numbers of entries in the Oxford Book of Quotations). It might be thought that because doctors and nurses have more frequent and closer encounters with death, they would be free of the constraints affecting the rest of society. This is not so. Many writers record the comments of dying patients who say that once the medical profession has admitted, to themselves, that cure is impossible, then they pass them by. Nurses, because of the nature of their role, continue to provide physical care but avoid anything but superficial conversation with the dying patient, apparently afraid of questions they will be unable to answer.

The bereaved frequently comment on their isolation. Friends either avoiding face-to-face encounters, or, if forced into conversation, refuse to discuss the topic uppermost in their minds, the death of the loved one.

Nurses are not only the people who have most contact with the dying, but they may be the first to talk to the recently bereaved, and therefore are frequently placed in the situation that society finds so difficult to cope with. The nurse herself may have a sense of failure in that a patient has died, and of loss, particularly when the deceased was well known and cared for over a long period.

Of course, nurses also have their own philosophies of life and death and these may or may not coincide with those held by the patient or the bereaved. Even if they are known, which is unlikely, the I.C.N. Code for Nurses states that 'the nurse, in providing care, promotes an environment in which the values, customs and spiritual beliefs of the individual are respected'. Yet, if beliefs are worth anything, they must affect the whole life of the individual and therefore influence the way that death is viewed. Not only that, if such beliefs hold hope and comfort for the individual, there will be a natural desire to share them so that the person in need can also be helped. The Christian nurse, in particular, may feel that she has an obligation to try to pass on this message to the dying patient, or the recently bereaved, while the non-Christian nurse may under-estimate the strength derived by the committed Christian patient from his relationship with God. The refusal of the Jehovah's witness to have the life-giving pint of blood, or the Orthodox Jew's rites for the dead may appear illogical to those whose belief is different.

What should be the approach of the nurse to the dying patient or his relatives? Unfortunately, many behave in the same way as the majority of the general population. They ignore the fact of death and never allow a conversation to develop.

A more difficult, but more useful approach is for the nurse to allow herself to get near to the dying patient, or the bereaved relatives, and allow him to talk. Such talking may include questions such as 'Why me?' 'What have I done wrong?' and so on, but these questions rarely require an answer. What they do need is a sympathetic listener. After the questions, the person may try to give explanations, often apportioning blame such as 'it would never have happened if I'd . . . '. This also requires little comment. Finally, statements may follow indicating a degree of acceptance of the situation. During this conversation, which may in fact be more of a monologue, the nurse may feel that she should put in words of explanation and examination, or cut short a distressing encounter. Such activity will prevent the working through of the stages of denial, blame and acceptance which are a necessary part of grieving for either one's own life in the case of the dying patient, or for the loss of a loved one. Only when this sequence has been accomplished is the nurse likely to be asked about her own beliefs in life, death and the life hereafter, and only then if her attitude has indicated that she has a positive contribution to make.

While in no way wishing to undermine the beliefs held by the nurse, guidance should be given on the way so that she may structure her role according to the various codes of ethics and/or professional conduct. Some statements are based on moral assumptions related to what is understood as 'good' or, 'just', while others may be more accurately called rules of etiquette in that they specify behaviour which may be morally neutral but which enable the smooth running of the organization to be carried out, or remind nurses of expected standards of conduct in a given culture. Yet other statements may be seen as guides to behaviour related to the protection of the public. Finally, some statements may be required to ensure the 'purity' of the profession.

The United Kingdom Central Council for Nursing, Midwifery and Health Visiting has recently issued a revised *Code of Professional Conduct for the Nurse, Midwife and Health Visitor* in which it clearly states that the main requirements are that 'each registered nurse, midwife and health visitor shall act, at all times, in such a manner as to justify public trust and confidence, to uphold and enhance the good standing and reputation of the profession, to sense the interests of society and ABOVE ALL safeguard the interests of individual patients and clients'.

The International Council for Nurses *Code for Nurses* also states that 'the prime responsibility of the nurse is the patient.' This centrality of accountability both for patient/client care, and to the patient/client for action, arises from the fundamental assumption that each individual is of equal worth. Such an assumption then precludes any discrimination in care regardless of class, creed or colour.

Probably all would agree with this fundamental view of the required actions of nursing. The conflict arises when a choice may have to be made between equal, but mutually exclusive claims. Some decisions may be medical not nursing decisions. (eg, the life of the mother or the baby). Others, especially those regarding resource allocation, may be administrative and, at the final point, practical (eg, more money for heart transplants or better resources for the care of the elderly). While it is comfortable to say that the decision in such cases does not rest with the nurse, she is still likely to be involved in the implications of such decisions and, as a member of society and an elector, she cannot absolve herself from the decision-making. Indeed, it may be in this situation that the role of the nurse as the patient's advocate (more easily depicted as companion or friend) has the major implications.

It is easy for the nurse to 'go with the crowd'. This is not merely unprofessional, but frequently verges on the immoral. Each nurse must decide on the basis of her actions and then abide by the implications. As discussed, if life is sacred, then procured abortion and euthanasia are not to be tolerated. If the one is acceptable, why not the other?

Such decisions are painful and often avoided. Nevertheless, they are basic to the way in which the nurse will react when confronted with certain aspects of patient care. This needs to be acknowledged by both the nurse and management, and the opportunity to make objections on the grounds of conscience to involvement in certain cases both offered and, if taken up, understood. Needless to say, the nurse must make such objections known to management before involvement is requested so that no patient is left without care.

Conflict may also arise when other members of the health care team view lines of treatment and care differently from the individual nurse. While in no way wishing to undermine the idea of cooperation with, and support of, colleagues, it is quite clear that the nurse's prime responsibility is to the patient. It is this type of discussion and perception of role in care that has not received much attention from nurse theorists and is therefore an area for research.

Many nursing theories have to date received little verification in the UK by the action of nurse researchers. All of them are based on idealised perceptions of nursing. There is nothing wrong in this approach, but practical application of these theories is required so that they can be tested in the organizational and environmental setting of nursing 'as it is'. Perhaps this book will stimulate such testing and lead to theories which are well validated or, if necessary, amended.

References and Further Reading

United Kingdom Central Council (1984) *Code of Professional Conduct for the Nurse, Midwife and Health Visitor*, 2nd edn UKCC, London

International Council of Nurses (1973) *Code for Nurses* ICN, Geneva
The codes denoted here are designed to help the nurse in carrying out nursing care by stating her duties and areas of accountability.
International Council of Nurses (1969) *Policy Statements.* ICN, Geneva
The policy statements denoted here are a series of statements covering specific situations, eg, the role of the nurse in the care of detainees and prisoners.

GLOSSARY

Abstract Related to ideas, not concrete.
Adaption All the activities a person may use to enable him to function as a person in society.
Altruistic Behaviour which is for the good of others.
Bias Weighting to one side. May be due to an individual's own values or preconceived ideas.
Concept An abstract idea.
Consensus Agreement.
Continuum A sequence of events. A continuous scale of characteristics used in measurement.
Convenience sample Items or people selected for testing because of their ease of access.
Correlation The relationship of two items. May be positive; that is, the two items will occur together and change together; or negative, as when item one increases the other item decreases.
Cultural lag The time taken for cultural change to spread throughout a given area or society.
Culture The norms, values, lifestyles of a specific society.

Cybernetics Self-regulatory control mechanisms.
Definition of the situation The interpretation or meaning given by an individual to the social situation in which he is placed.
Deviancy Behaviour outside the norms or limits set by a specific society.
Discrimination Distinguishing different groups of people or factors. Frequently used to indicate a different form of behaviour.
Egoistic Concerned with oneself. Selfish.
Elite The best. A superior group.
Empirical Information gained through the senses, or by experience.
Environment The constantly changing surroundings, comprising places, people, objects and, in certain cases, ideas.
Expressive Outward demonstration, usually related to feelings.
Homeostasis A term used to describe changes which occur in man to maintain balance. Used in sociology to indicate a self regulating mechanism in society.
Hypothesis A supposition made on the basis of reasoning. A statement to be tested.
Ideology A set of concepts and beliefs which are held to explain social phenomena, not necessarily true.
Intervention Specific action taken to alter the course of events
Labelling The process by which individuals may be categorized according to social behaviour or any other attribute. Diagnosis is an example of a specific type of labelling.
Model A conceptual framework capable of explaining or illustrating a complex situation. May be verbal, diagrammatic or mathematical.
Phenomenology The study of phenomen in society.
Profession A term applied to occupations which are able to demonstrate specific characteristics including specialized knowledge and skill, and autonomy of action.
Random sample Each item has equal chance of being selected.
Role The part an individual plays as a result of occupying some position in life.

Sanctions Adverse actions applied to an individual who does not adhere to society's norms.
Self concept image The individual's psychological view of himself.
Self-fulfilling prophecies Behaviour from an individual or group which develops as a result of the expectation of its development by others — originally absent.
Significance When used related to research, indicates whether or not the findings could have occurred by chance.
Social exchange The demands and rewards made and offered by individuals as they interact.
Stereotype A set image of an object, individual, group.
Stigma Imputation of an adverse type attached to an individual indicating that the person is not'normal'.
Stressor Any factor which requires an output of energy.
Symbolic interaction Interaction between people who define and interpret the meaning of each other's actions.
System Any organized body of action or material working in a coordinated manner.
Task allocation A nurse is usually given one or more tasks to carry out on all the patients requiring such attention, eg, all the pressure area care, all the mouth toilets.
Team Nursing A small number of nurses carrying out all the care for a small group of patients.
Theory A statement describing the relationship between phenomena or concepts which have been shown (by research) to exist. May be used to explain empirical findings.

INDEX OF NAMES

INDEX OF SUBJECTS